International Environmental Labelling

Vol.4 of 11
For All People who wish to take care of Climate Change
Health & Beauty Industries: (Fragrances, Makeup, Cosmetics,
Personal Care, Sunscreen, Toothpaste,
Bathing, Nailcare & Shaving, Skin Care, Foot Care, Hair Care
and Other Health & Beauty Products)

Jahangir Asadi

Vancouver, BC CANADA

Suggest an ecolabel

If you think that we missed a label and/or you are an ecolabelling body, please consider to submit for the next editions of our 11 Volumes International Eco-labelling Book series. Please send your details, and we'll review your suggestions. Our goal is to be as comprehensive as possible, so thank you for your help!

info@TopTenAward.Net

Published by: Top Ten Award International Network
Vancouver, BC **CANADA**
Email: Info@TopTenAward.net
www.TopTenAward.net

Ordering Information:
Quantity sales. Special discounts are available on quantity purchases by universities, schools, corporations, associations, and others. For details, contact the "Sales Department" at the above mentioned email address.

International Environmental Labelling Vol.4/J.Asadi—1st ed.
ISBN 978-1-7773356-6-3

Contents

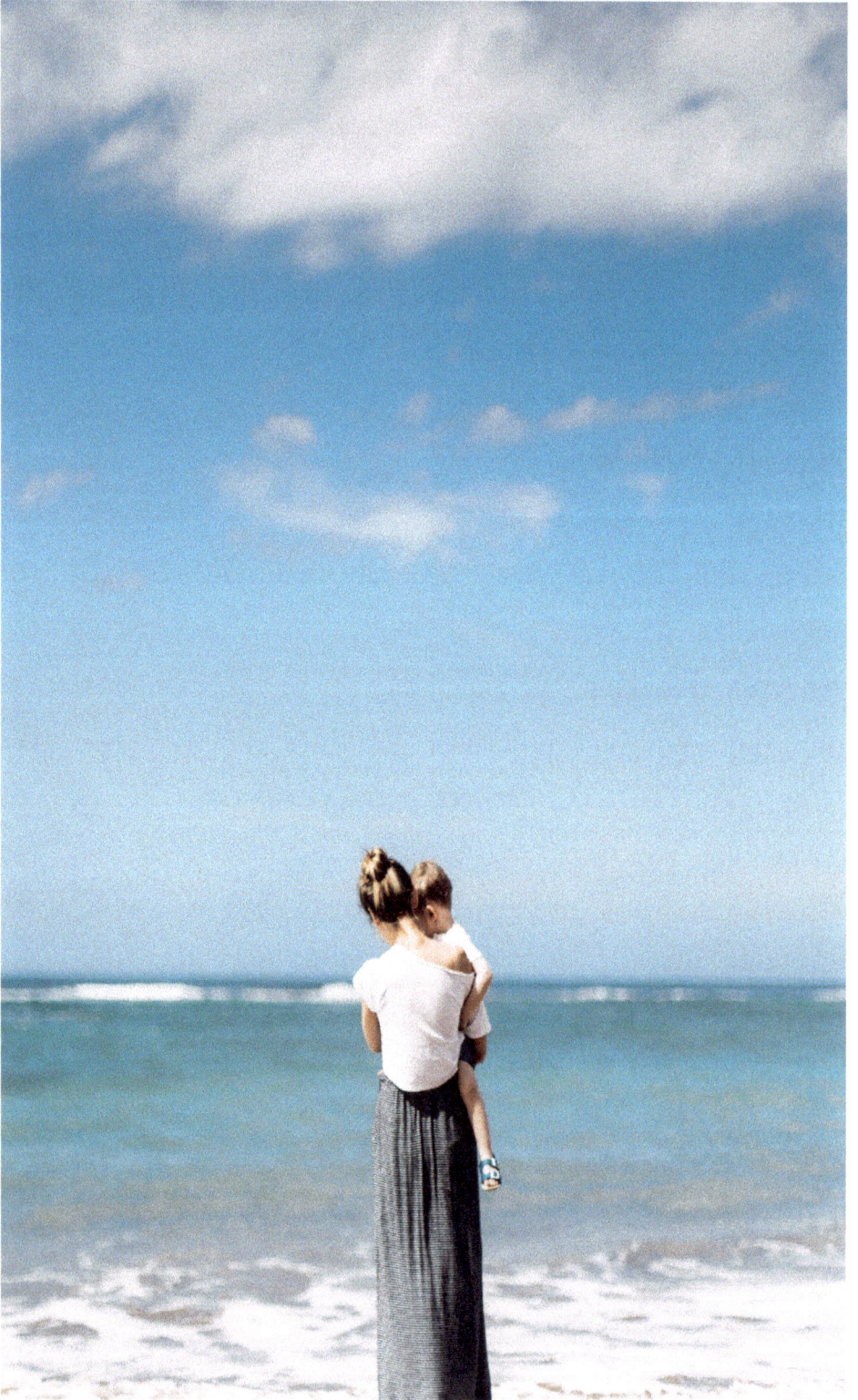

I dedicate this book to my Dad & Mum.

We hope that, 10,000 years from now, future generations will be able to see flowers that provide bees with nectar and pollen and... BEES provide flowers with the means to reproduce by spreading pollen from flower to flower...

Jahangir Asadi

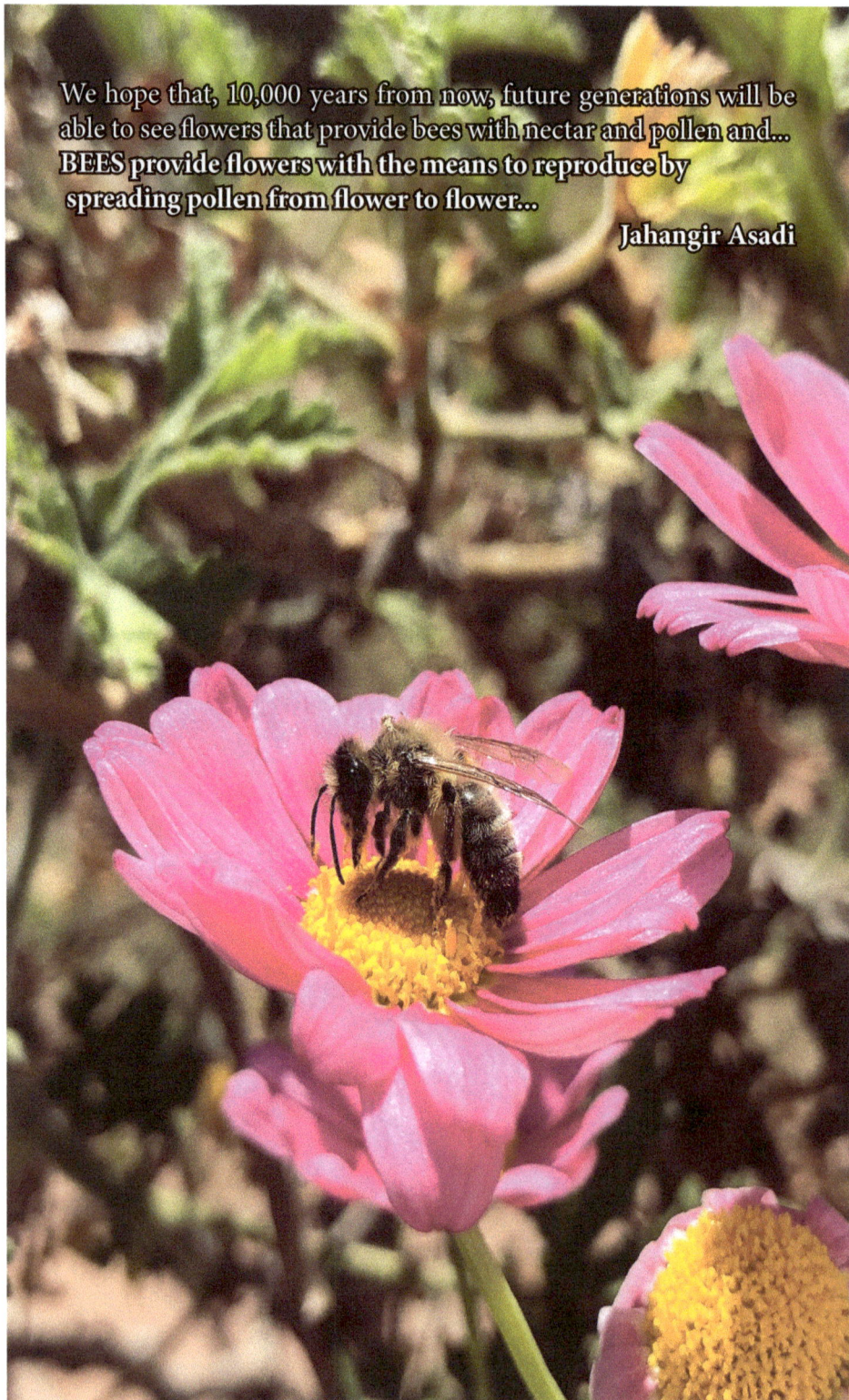

Acknowledgements:

I wish to thank my committee members, who were more than generous with their expertise and precious time. I would like to acknowledge and thank the Top Ten Award International Network for allowing me to conduct my research and providing any assistance requested.

It should be noted that all the required permissions for using the logos and trade marks has been obtained to be published in this volume.

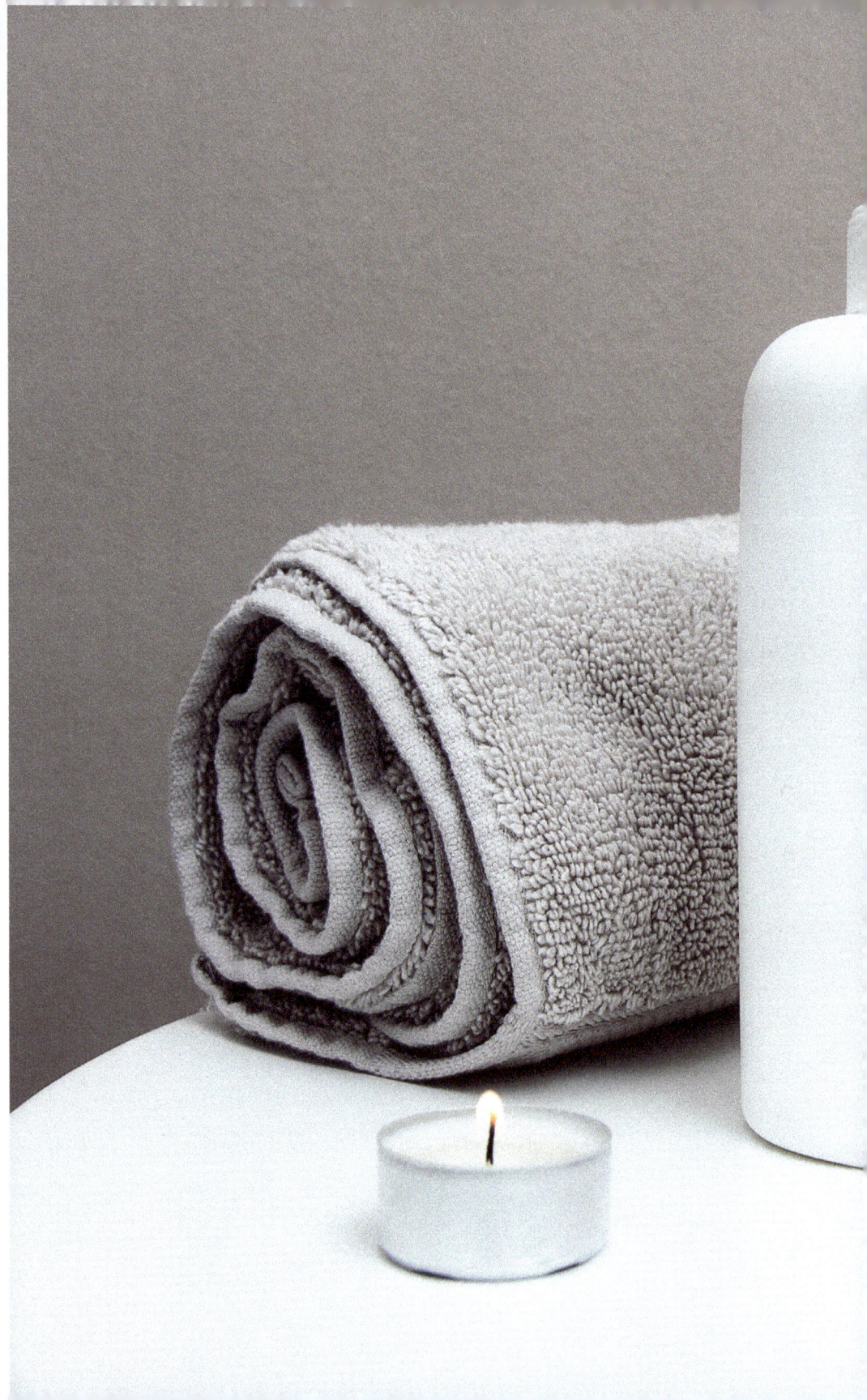

How your beauty products are affecting the environment?

Everything you use has an impact on the planet, including beauty products. The cosmetics and skincare industry is known for its heavy use of plastics, especially in their packaging. Plastic waste takes hundreds of years to decompose, and it often ends up getting stuck in landfills or eaten by animals.

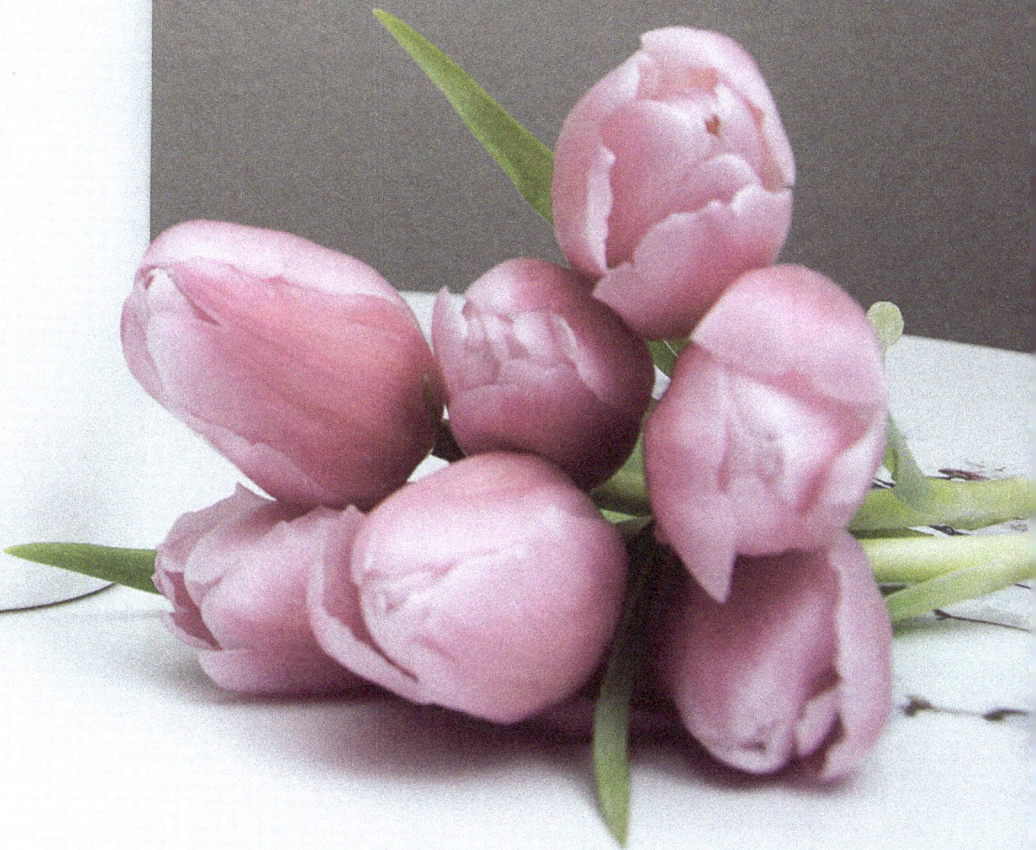

Top Ten Award International Network

Top Ten Award international Network (TTAIN) was established in 2012 to recognize outstanding individuals, groups, companies, organizations representing the best in the public works profession.

TTAIN publishing books related to international Eco-labeling plans to increase public knowledge in purchasing based on the environmental impacts of products.

Top Ten Award International Network provides A to Z book publishing services and distribution to over 39,000 booksellers worldwide, including Apple, Amazon, Barnes & Noble, Indigo, Google Play Books, and many more.

Our services including: editing, design, distribution, marketing

TTAIN Book publishing are in the following categories:

Student
Standard
Business
Professional
Honorary

We focus on quality, environmental & food safety management systems , as well as environmnetal sustain for future kids. TTAIN also provide complete consulting services for QMS, EMS, FSMS, HACCP and Ecolabeling based on international standards.

ISO 14024 establishes the principles and procedures for developing Type I environmental labelling programmes, including the selection of product categories, product environmental criteria and product function characteristics, and for assessing and demonstrating compliance. ISO 14024 also establishes the certification procedures for awarding the label.

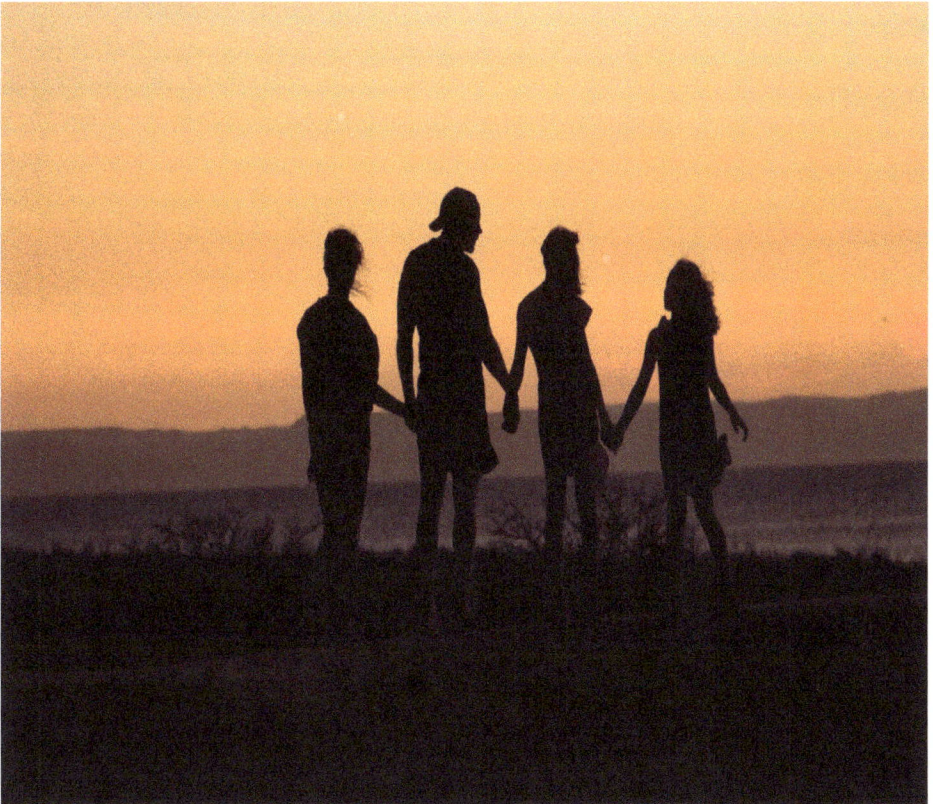

TTAIN has enough experiences to help create new ecolabeling programmes in different countries all over the world.
For more detail visit our website : http://toptenaward.net
and/or send your enquiery to the following email:
info@toptenaward.net

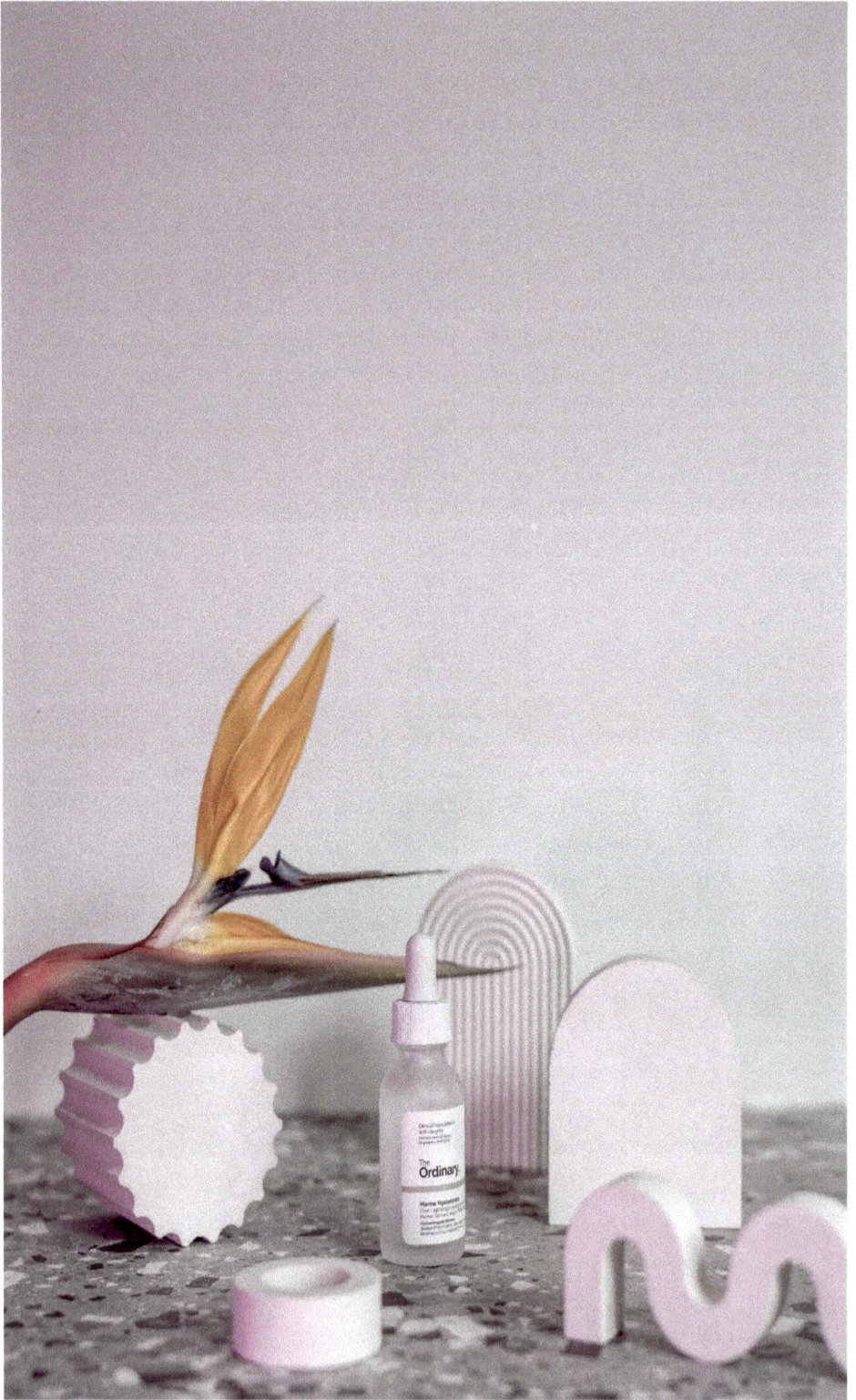

CHAPTER 1

Introduction

This book is dedicated to the subject of environmental labels. The basis for the classification of its parts goes back to the types of environmental labelling according to the classifications provided by the International Organization for Standardization. In each section, while presenting the relevant definitions, I mention the existing international standards and present examples related to each type of labelling. Environmental labelling is an important and significant topic, and its richness is added to every day, which has attracted the attention of many experts and researchers around the world. The idea of compiling this book, came to my mind when I observed that national environmental labelling models have been developed in most countries of the world, but in many other countries, the initial steps have not been taken yet. Therefore, I decided to create the first spark for the development of environmental labelling patterns in other countries by collecting appropriate materials and inserting samples of labelling patterns of different countries of the world. It should be noted that the description of each environmental label in this book does not indicate their approval or denial; they are included only to increase the awareness of all enthusiasts and consumers of the meanings and concepts derived from such labels. We hereby ask all interested parties around the world who wish to start an environmental labelling program in their country to benefit from our intellectual assistance and support in the form of consulting contracts. Increasing human awareness of the urgent need to protect the environment has led to changes in all levels of activities, including the production of marketing products, consumption, use, and sale of goods and services at the national and international levels. Stakeholders involved in environmental protection include consumers, producers, traders, scientific and technological institutes, national authorities, local and international organizations, environmental gatherings, and human society in general. Decisions by consumers and sellers of products are made not only on the basis of key points such as quality, price, and availability of

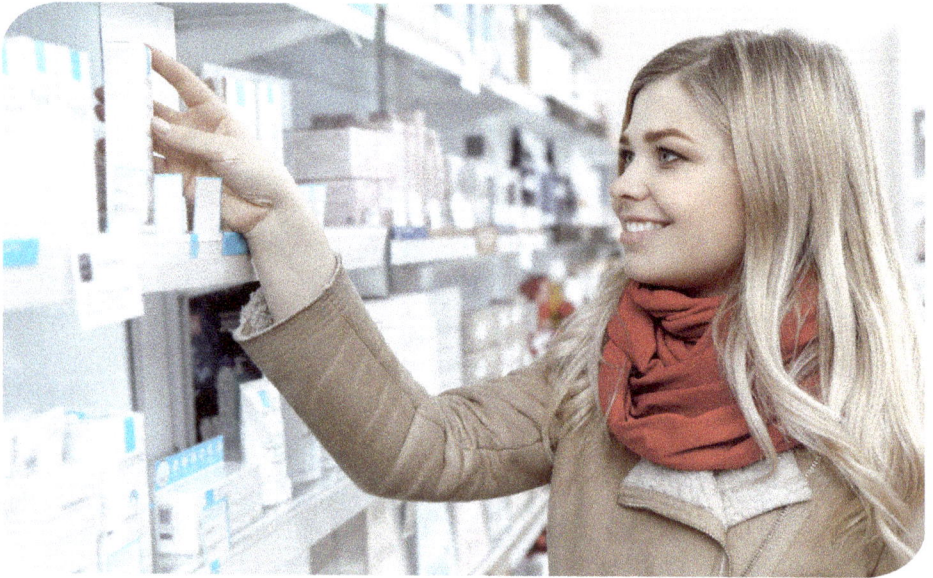

products but also on the environmental consequences of products, including the consequences that a product can have before, after and during production. The most important environmental consequences include water, soil, and air pollution along with waste generation, especially hazardous waste. Further consequences include noise, odor, dust, vibration, and heat dissipation as well as energy consumption using water, land, fuel, wood, and other natural resources. There are further effects on certain parts of the ecosystem and the environment. In addition, the environmental consequences not only include the natural use of the products but also abnormal and even emergency or accidental uses. The basis of studies and studies in this field is done through product life cycle evaluation, which generally involves the study and evaluation of environmental aspects and consequences of a category (product, service, etc.) because of the preparation of raw materials for production until they are used or discarded. Sometimes the phrase "review from cradle to grave" is used for such an evaluation. In addition to the above, the environmental consequences that may occur at any stage of the product life cycle, including the preliminary stages and its preparation, production, distribution, operation, and sale, should also be considered when evaluating it. This type of evaluation refers to product life cycle analysis from an environmental point of view,"

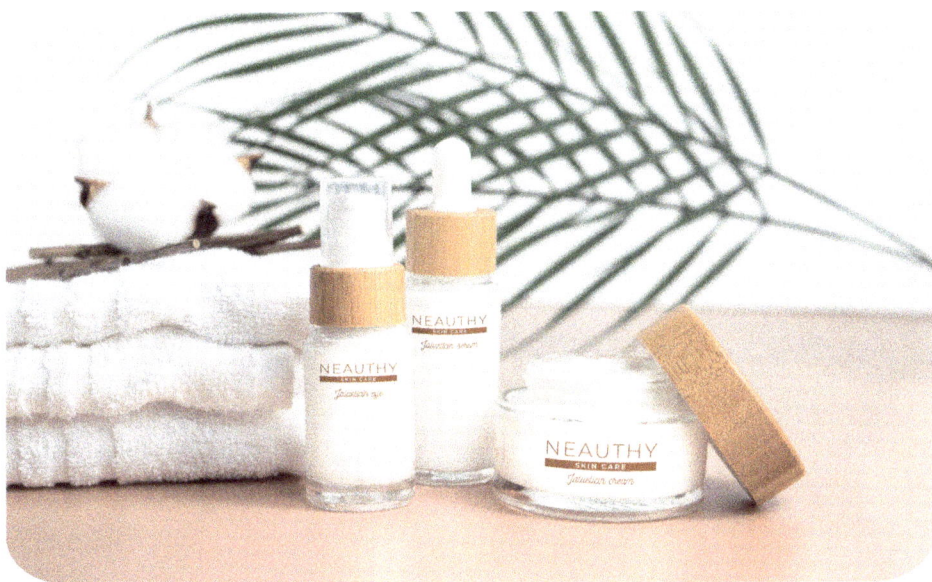

which is a useful tool for measuring the degree of environmental health of a product, comparing different products, improving product quality, and confirming the environmental health claims of the product. The environmental health analysis tool for products and services facilitates their placement in domestic or foreign markets, considering that the awareness of consumers and retailers about the environmental consequences of the product has increased, as has the accurate and explicit measurement by the people in charge at all levels. Local, national, and international in the field of environmental protection. Products that can claim to be environ-

mentally complete in all stages of their life cycle and meet the mandato-
ry and optional environmental needs are considered successful products.
Environmental messages refer to the policies, goals, and skills of product
manufacturing companies as part of the environmental management systems in which they are applied, and consumers and retailers are increasingly paying attention to this issue when making purchasing decisions. In
addition, companies have been encouraged and even forced to adapt their
environmental management systems to agencies and retailers and to local,
national, international, and other environmental issues.

The environmental health message of a product can be conveyed to the
consumer in various ways, including implicitly or explicitly. For example,
the implicit or implicit message conveyed directly by the product to the
customer is that the product is suitable for the intended use and purpose,
and, without material waste in size, weight, and dimensions, is perfectly
proportioned and without additional packaging. Sometimes it is necessary
to convey these messages and claims about the correctness of the product
quite clearly through magazines or other media as well as through certificates that are accurate, simple, and convincing to the consumer in the
form of a label. These messages must be accurate and fact-based; other-
wise they will nullify the product and create contradictory effects. Con-
firmation of these claims by a third-party organization will increase its
credibility. It should also be noted that the multiplicity of these messages,
depending on the type of products or companies producing them, confuses
consumers in the market and also creates artificial boundaries or causes a
differentiated distinction against certain products or companies. Various
models, principles, and methods have been provided by local, regional,
national, and international organizations to demonstrate product life cycle
analysis and other guidelines on environmental management systems and
their labels. At the national level, significant advances have been made
in the design of environmental labels in various countries, including developing countries and the Scandinavian countries. For example, the first
project was designated in Germany as a Blue Angel in 1977, later on Canada in 1988, the Scandinavian countries and Japan in 1989, the United
States and New Zealand in 1990, India, Austria, and Australia in 1991,
And in 1992, Singapore, the Republic of Korea, and the Netherlands de-

veloped their national environmental labelling. Environmental labels are an environmental management tool that is the subject of a series of ISO 14000 standards. These environmental labels provide information about a product or commodity in terms of its broad environmental characteristics, whether it is about a specific environmental issue or about other characteristics and topics.Interested and pro-environmental buyers can use this information when choosing products or goods. Product makers with these environmental labels hope to influence people's purchasing decisions. If these environmental labels have this effect, the share of the product in question can increase, and other suppliers may create healthy environmental competition by improving the environmental aspects of their products and commodities. The overall goal of environmental labels is to convey acceptable and accurate information that is in no way misleading regarding the environmental aspects of products and commodities, and they encourage the consumer to buy and produce products that reduce stress on the environment. Environmental labelling must follow the general principles that the International Organization for Standardization has published in a collection entitled the ISO 14020 standard, which refers to these general principles here. It should be noted that other documents and laws in this field are considered if they are in accordance with the principles set out in ISO 14020.

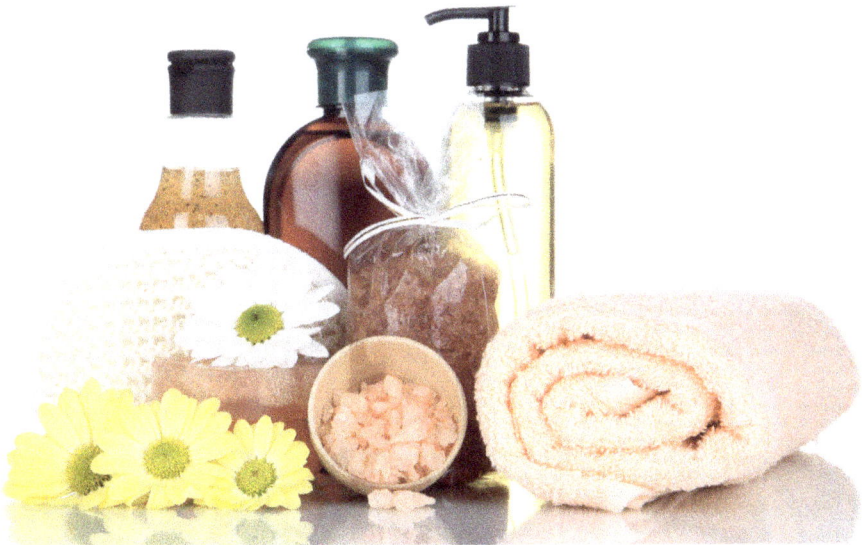

WATER OIL
SKIN P...

SONIA ROSELLI

Fragrance Free

1.52 fl oz (45ml)

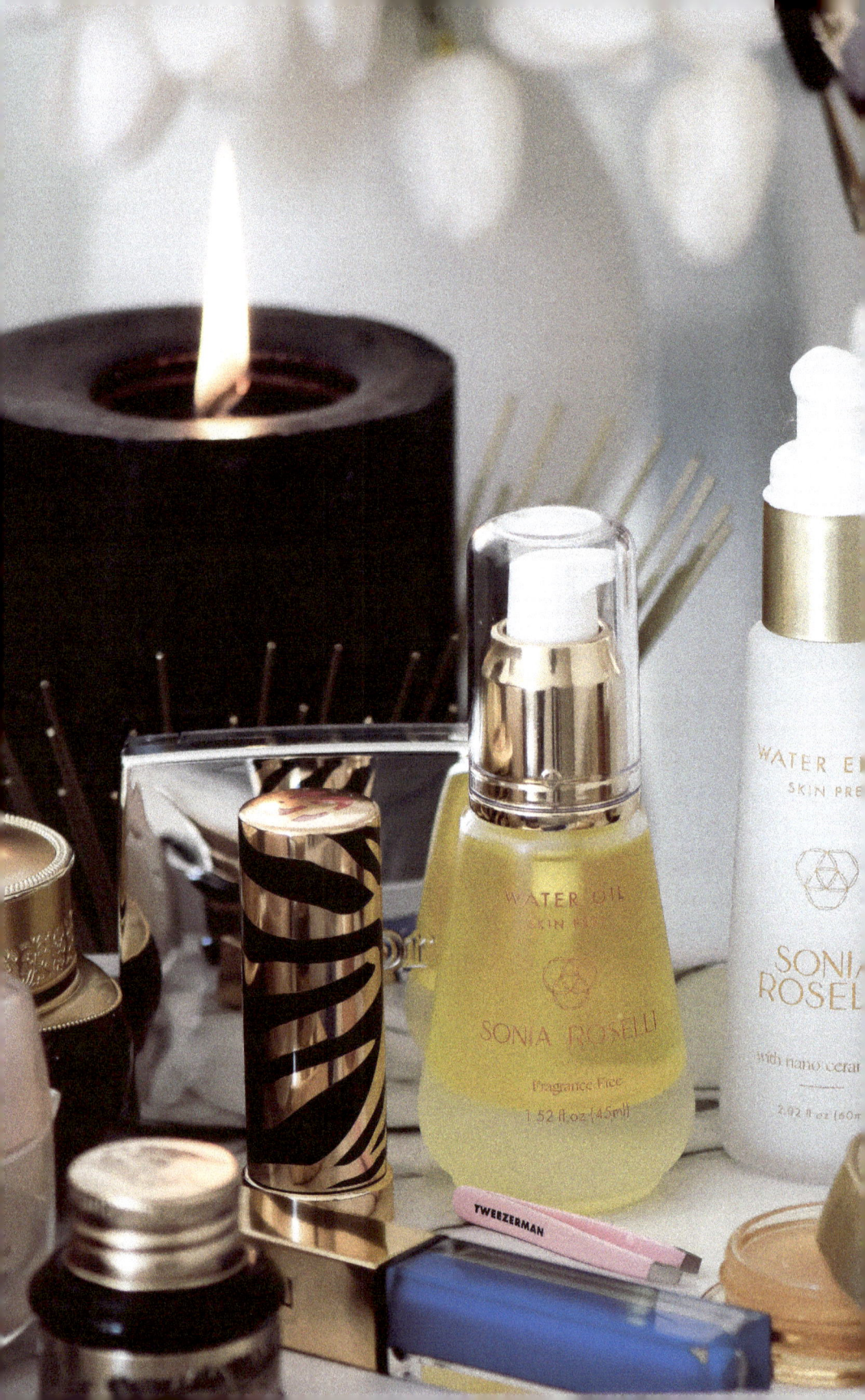

WATER EL...
SKIN PRE...

SONIA
ROSEL...

with nano ceram...

2.02 fl oz (60...

TWEEZERMAN

The purchase process of natural cosmetics is influenced by the presence of eco-labels, which informs the consumer about the impact on environment and health. Due to the popularity of natural cosmetics with an eco-label, a growing amount of companies use eco-labels on their packaging.

CHAPTER **2**

General Principles on Environmental Labelling

1 The First Principle: Evironmental notices and labels must be accurate, verifiable, relevant, and in no way misleading and/or deceptive.

2 The Second Principle: Procedures and requirements for environmental labels will not be ready for selection unless they are implemented by affecting or eliminating unnecessary barriers to international trade.

3 The Third Principle: Environmental notices and labels will be based on scientific analysis that is sufficiently broad and comprehensive, and to support this claim, the product must be reliable and reproducible.

4 The Fourth Principle: The process, methodology, and any criteria required to support the announcements on environmental labels will be available upon request all interested groups.

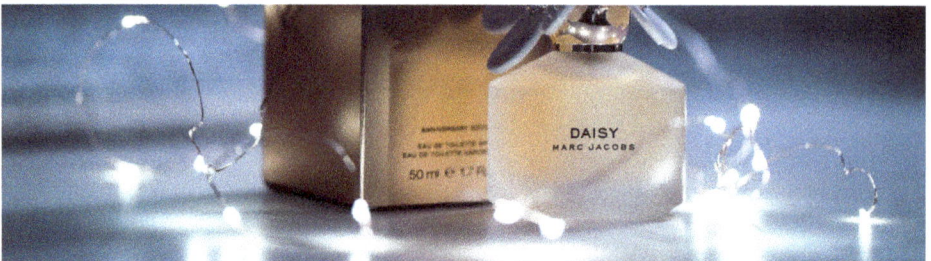

5 The Fifth Principle: Development and improvement of environmental notices and labels should be considered in all aspects related to the service life of the product.

6 The Sixth Principle: Announcements on environmental labels will not prevent initiative and innovation but will be important in maintaining environmental implementation.

7 The Seventh Principle: Any enforcement request or information requirement related to environmental notices and labels should be limited to the necessary information to establish compliance with an acceptable standard and based on the notification standards and environmental labels.

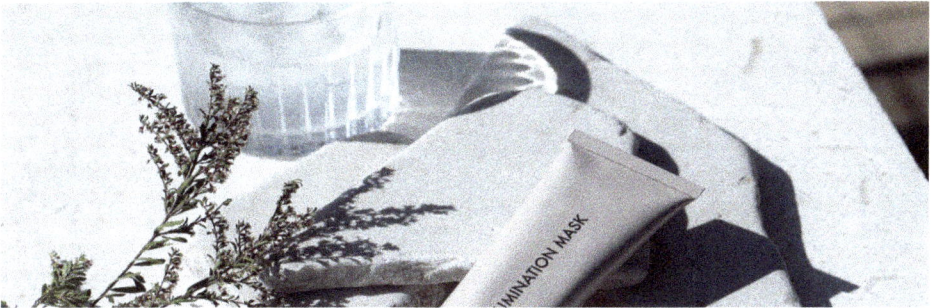

8 The Eighth Principle: The process of improving the announcement and environmental labels should be done by an open solution with interested groups. Reasonable impressions must be made to reach a consensus through this process.

9 The Ninth Principle: Information on the environmental aspects of the product and goods related to an advertisement and environmental label will be prepared for buyers and interested buyers from a group consisting of an advertisement and an environmental label.

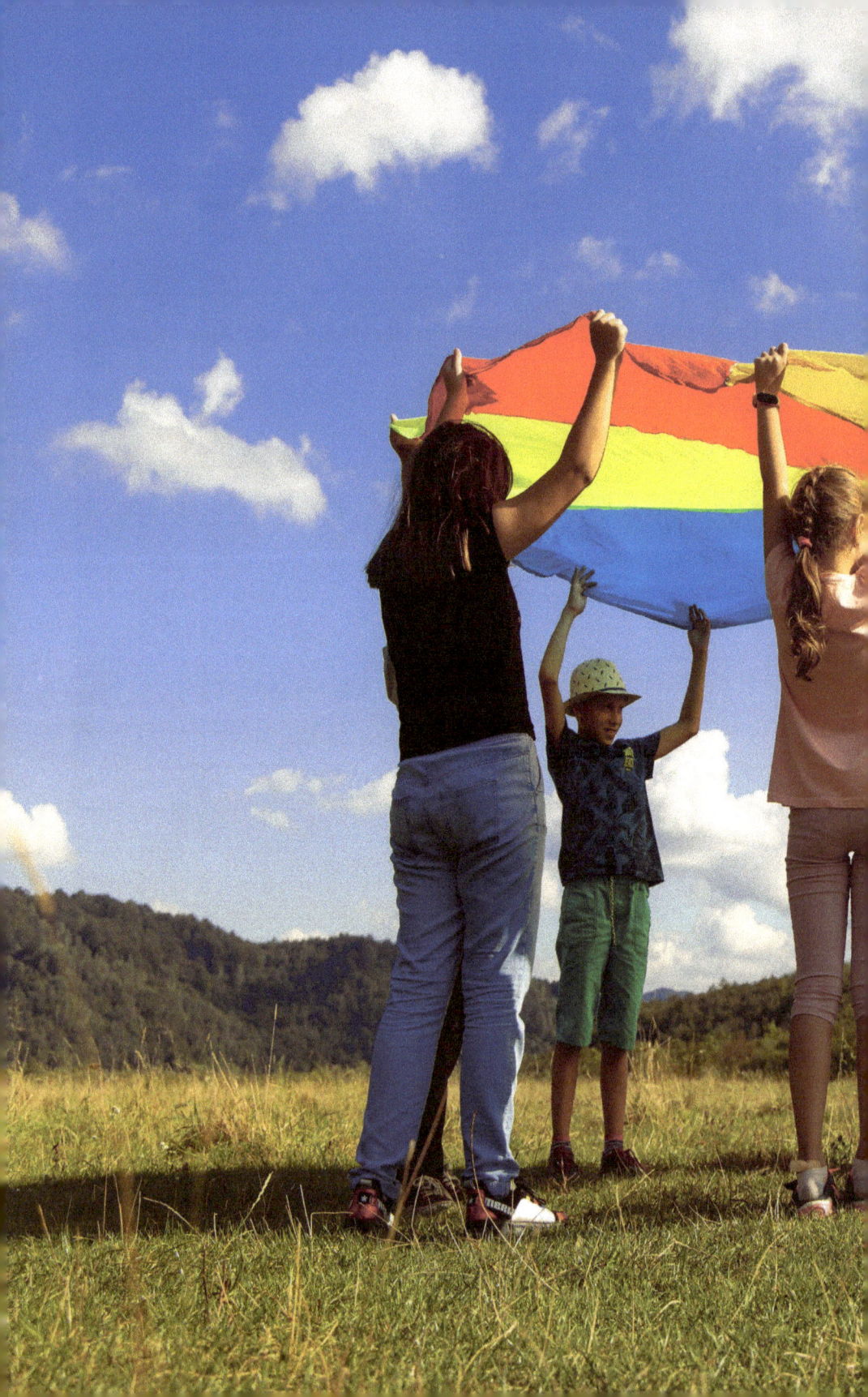

Eco-labels inform consumers about the environmental influence of a specific product. The purchase intention for eco-labelled cosmetics is positively influenced by the understanding of eco-labels, attention for eco-labels and product preference for eco-labelled products.

CHAPTER 3

Types of Environmental Labelling

At present, according to the classification provided by the International Organization for Standardization, there are three types of environmental labelling patterns:

1 Type I labelling: This labelling is known as eco-labelling, and because it is difficult to translate this word into many languages, it presents another reason to adhere to a numerical classification system. In the content of Type I labelling, a set of social commitments that creates criteria according to the scientific principles on the basis of which a product is environmentally preferable is discussed. Consumers are then instructed in assessing environmental claims and must decide which packaging is more important.

2 Type II labelling: refers to the claims made on product labels in connection with business centers. This includes familiar claims such as recyclable, ozone-friendly, 60% phosphate-free, and the like. This type of labelling can be in the form of a mark or sentence on the product packaging. Some of them are valid environmental claims—and some can be completely misleading. Usually, all countries have laws against deceptive advertisements, so why has the International Organization for Standardization discussed this issue? The answer is that it is not clear whether the environmental claims have a technical basis or whether the ad is meaningless.

3 Type III labelling: is a distinct form of third-party environmental labelling pattern designed to avoid the difficulties that can result from type-one labelling. Technical committee for Environment of International organization for Standardization has undertaken a new project to standardize guidelines and Type III labelling methods. One of the main objections raised by industries to Type I labelling is the basis for its management.

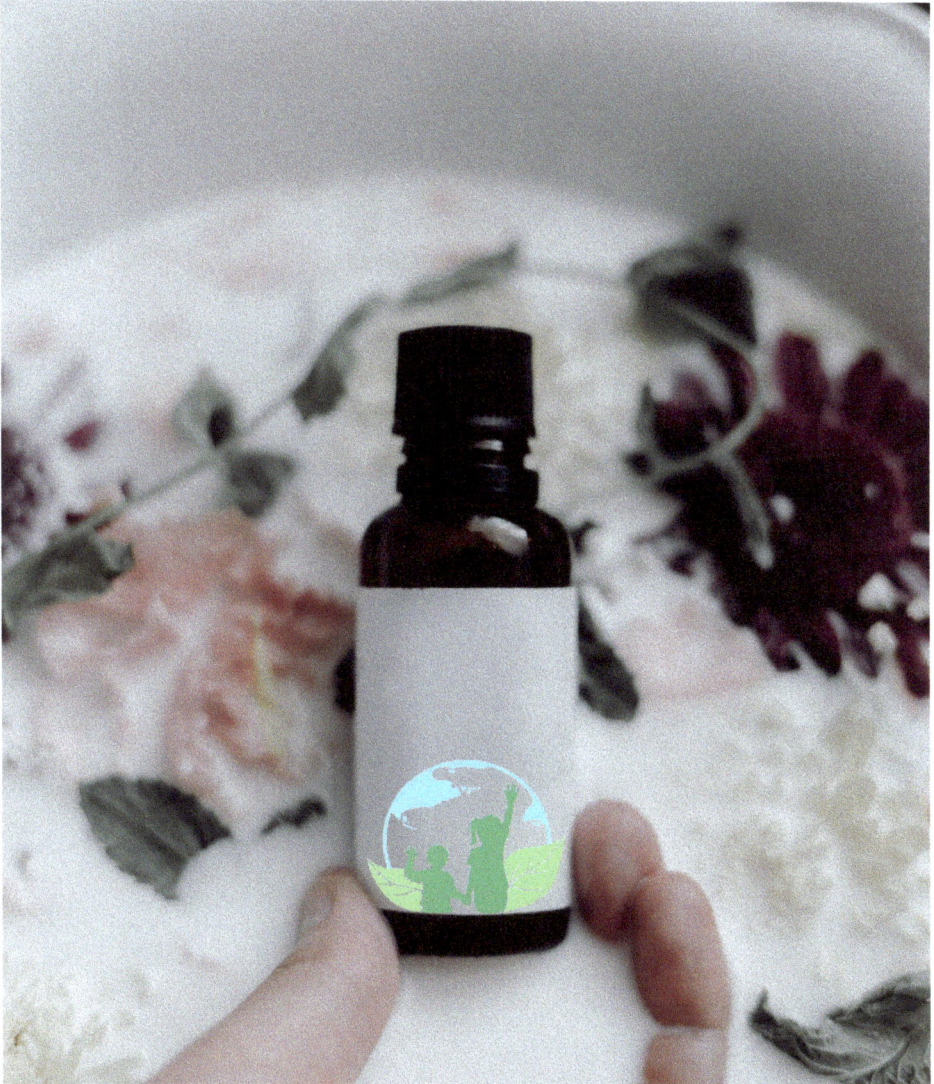

What is meant by vegan cosmetics?
When a beauty product is marked as vegan, it means the same thing a vegan diet does. This label infers that the product does not contain any animal or its byproducts in it.

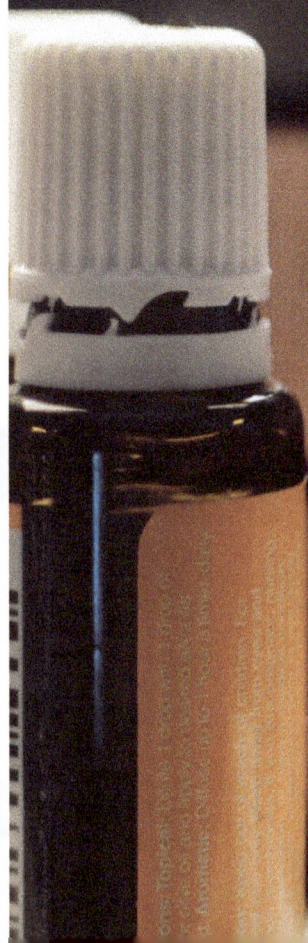

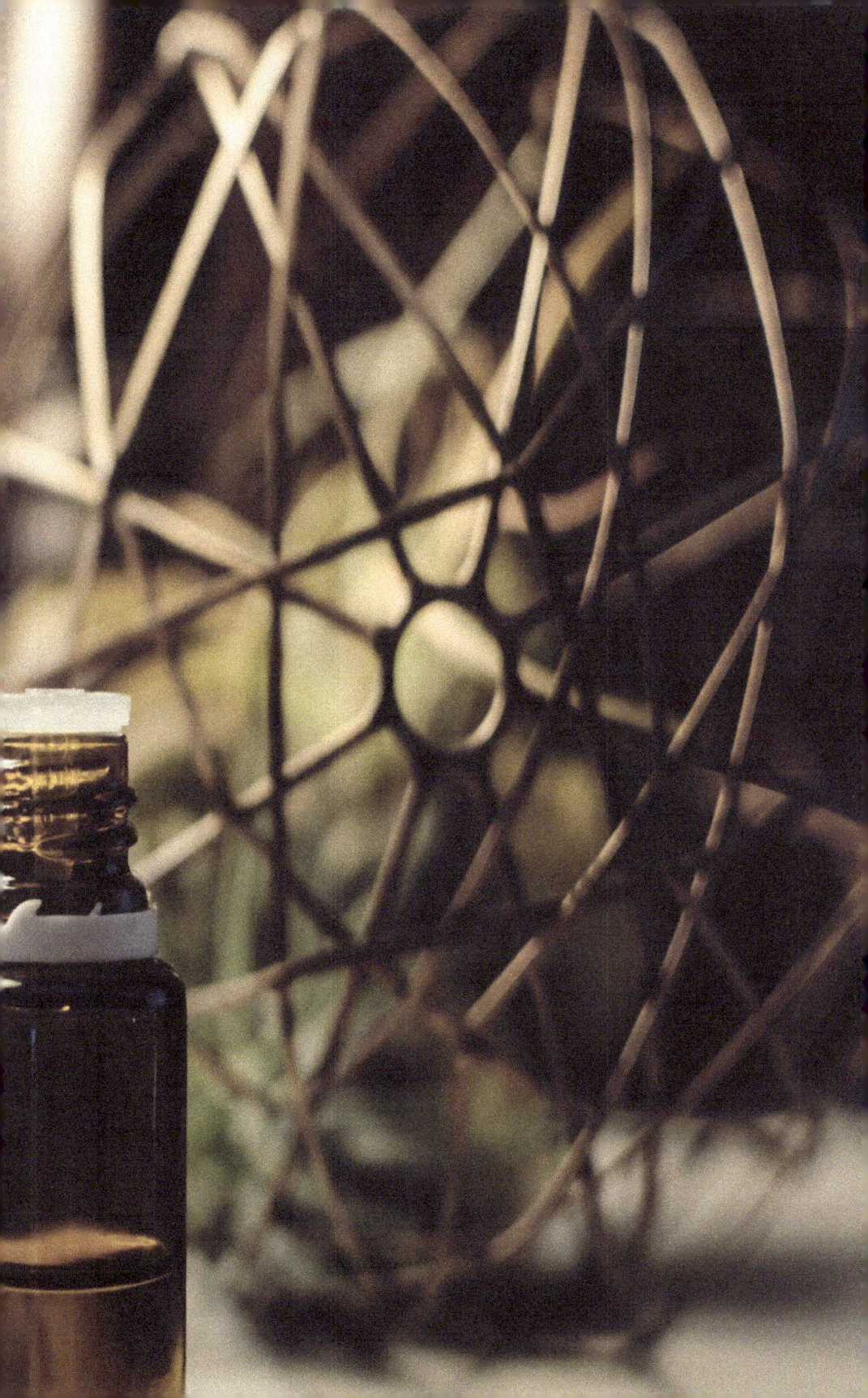

CHAPTER 4

Type I Environmental Labelling

Type I labelling: This labelling is known as eco-labelling, and because it is difficult to translate this word into many languages, it presents another reason to adhere to a numerical classification system. In the content of Type I labelling, a set of social commitments that creates criteria according to the scientific principles on the basis of which a product is environmentally preferable is discussed. Consumers are then instructed in assessing environmental claims and must decide which packaging is more important.

Type I adhesive has the following specifications:
A. Has an optional third-party template.
B. When the product meets a certain standard, the labelling of this product is included.
C. The purpose of this program is to identify and promote products that play a pioneering role in terms of environment, which means its criteria are at a higher level than the average environmental performance.
D. Acceptance/rejection criteria are determined for each group of products and are publicly available.
E. The criteria are adjusted after considering the environmental consequences of the product life cycle.

Examples of Type I Labelling:
In this section, and considering the importance of this type of labelling, I provide a description of some examples of Type I labelling related to some countries along with a   list of products on which this mark is placed.

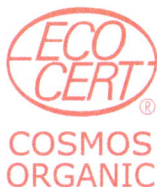

COSMOS
ORGANIC

Global

Certification against the international COSMOS-Standard will enable you to label your product as "natural" or "organic."

All products marketed with the ECOCERT logo have been verified by our teams: from composition to processing and packaging. Consumers are thus given transparent information on the content of natural and organic ingredients that are listed on the product label.

Requirements for labeling:

Natural origin

All the ingredients are derived from natural origin except those included in a restrictive approved ingredients list (including preservatives) which are authorized in small quantities.

In general, ECOCERT certifies products as "natural" if they contain at least 95% ingredients of natural origin.

Promoting Organic

A beauty care product may be COSMOS ORGANIC certified only if:
• At least 95% of the ingredients are of natural origin,
• At least 95% of all ingredients that can be sourced as organic, must be organic
• At least 20% organic ingredients in the product (10% for rinse-off products and powders).

Contact:

Web: https://www.ecocert.com/en-CA/
Tel.: (+1) 418-838-6941

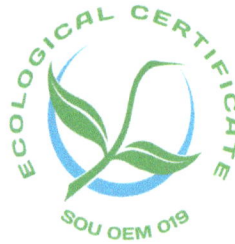

Ukraine

The ecolabelling program in Ukraine was founded on the initiative of the All-Ukrainian NGO "Living Planet" in 2003. The Green Crane is the first and the only one Type 1 Ecolabel in Ukraine that recognized officially.

The main objective of company's activity is to evaluate the products for compliance with environmental criteria according to ISO 14024 scheme in order to ensure the reliability of data on the environmental benefits of products within a specific category based on the results of the life cycle assessment. Over the 16 years of the program's existence, the Green Crane ecolabel has become a recognizable reliable reference point for consumers and government organizations (in "green procurement" process), as well as effective marketing tool for business.

Program Statistical Information. Today, the program operates with 57 certification standarts in various industries - construction, food, chemical, textile and other. More than 500 certificates have been issued throughout the program's history. Currently, 68 certificates for more than 1,000 products are valid.

Contact:
NGO «Living Planet»
Email: os@ecolabel.org.ua,
             info@ecolabel.org.ua
Tel: +380 44 332 84 08
Adress: Magnitogorsky Lane1-B, Kyiv, Ukraine - 02094
Web: https://www.ecolabel.org.ua/en

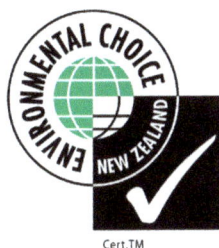

New Zealand

Environmental Choice New Zealand (ECNZ) is the country›s only Government-owned ecolabel. Administered by the New Zealand Ecolabelling Trust, the ecolabel was established in 1992 to provide a credible and independent guide for businesses and consumers to purchase and use products that are better for the environment.

A member of the Global Ecolabelling Network, ECNZ is a Type I ecolabel, which means products and services bearing the label meet criteria covering the whole life-cycle of the product/service, from raw materials, through manufacture and usage, to end-of-life disposal or reuse. Licensed products and services are independently assessed regularly by a third party.

The New Zealand Ecolabelling Trust
PO Box 56 533, Dominion Rd, Mt Eden, Auckland 1446
Tel: 0064 9 845 3330
Email: info@environmentalchoice.org.nz
Web: www.environmentalchoice.org.nz

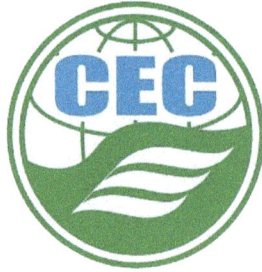

China

China Environmental United Certification Center (CEC), approved by the Ministry of Ecology and Environment of the People's Republic of China (MEE) and accredited by Certification and Accreditation Administration Committee of PRC, is a comprehensive certification and service institution leading in environmental protection, energy saving and low carbon areas. . CEC is committed to serve building national ecological civilization; and has carried out research on environmental protection, energy saving, low carbon development strategies and solutions; has been continuously improving and innovating green industry evaluation system on industrial green development and transition CEC is building a bridge between green production and green consumption by offering independent, impartial and high-quality evaluation and certification service for government, enterprises and the public. CEC is a state-owned, non-profit, legal entity of independent third-party certification. It integrates the certification resource from the former National Accreditation Center for Environmental Conformity Assessment, the Secretariat of China Environmental Labelling Products Certification Committee, Environmental Development Center of MEE, the Chinese Research Academy of Environmental Sciences and other institutions. Business areas includes: products certification, management systems certification, services certification, addressing climate change, energy-saving and energy efficiency certification, green supply chain assessment, environmental stewardship, green credit assessment and green manufacturing system evaluation. CEC also carries out standard establishment and research project and international cooperation and exchanges, etc.

Contact:
Website: http://en.mepcec.com/
E-mail: zhangxiaoh@mepcec.com , zhangxiaoh@mepcec.com

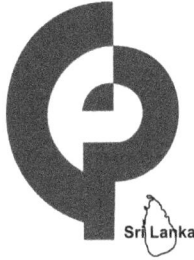

Sri Lanka

Sri Lanka

National Cleaner Production Centre (NCPC), Sri Lanka was set up by UNIDO in 2002, as a project under the Ministry of Industry to provide the technical expertise and support to the industry and business enterprises in order to prevent pollution and conserve resources by the application of Cleaner Production (CP) and other proactive environmental management tools. NCPC Sri Lanka is registered as a Company by Guarantee not for profit organization under the Act No. 7 of 2007. Over the past two decades, it has evolved as the foremost sustainability solution provider in the country.

The ISO 9001:2015 certified Centre is a registered Energy Service Company (ESCO) under Sustainable Energy Authority (SEA) and a registered consultant under Central Environmental Authority (CEA). It is a founding member of UNIDO/UNEP Resource Efficient and Cleaner Production Network (RECP Net), a global family of 52 NCPCs. NCPC Sri Lanka is a member of Climate Technology Centre & Network (CTCN) and associate member of Global Eco-labelling Network (GEN). Accordingly, we at National Cleaner Production Centre (NCPC), Sri Lanka has developed Eco Labelling scheme under the ISO 14024:2018 - Environmental labels and declarations. NCPC Eco labelling scheme developed, with the Support of United Nations Environment Programme, Under One Planet Network Consumer Information Programme for Sustainable Consumption and Production (CI-SCP).

Contact:
Tel: +94 11 2822272/3,
Fax: +94 11 2822274
E mail: info@ncpcsrilanka.org
Web: www.ncpcsrilanka.org

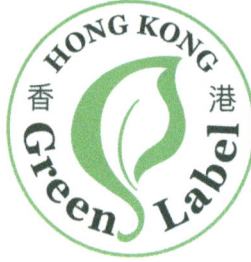

Hong Kong

The Green Council is a non-profit, tax-exempt charitable environmental stewardship organisation and certification body (Reg. No.: HKCAS-027) of Hong Kong established in 2000. A group of individuals from different sectors of industry and academics shared the vision to help build Hong Kong into a world-class green city for the future. They formed the Green Council with the aim of encouraging the commercial and industrial sectors to include environmental protection in their management and production processes. The Green Council is a non-profit, tax-exempt charitable environmental stewardship organisation and certification body (Reg. No.: HKCAS-027) of Hong Kong established in 2000. A group of individuals from different sectors of industry and academics shared the vision to help build Hong Kong into a world-class green city for the future. They formed the Green Council with the aim of encouraging the commercial and industrial sectors to include environmental protection in their management and production processes. The Green Council is a non-profit, tax-exempt charitable environmental stewardship organisation and certification body (Reg. No.: HKCAS-027) of Hong Kong established in 2000. A group of individuals from different sectors of industry and academics shared the vision to help build Hong Kong into a world-class green city for the future. They formed the Green Council with the aim of encouraging the commercial and industrial sectors to include environmental protection in their management and production processes.

Contact:
Website: https://www.greencouncil.org/hkgls
Email: info@greencouncil.org
Telephone: (852) 2810 1122

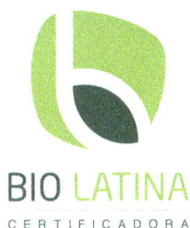

Peru

BIO LATINA, the consolidated byproduct of four Latin American national certification entities.Since 1998, we have provided certification services in Latin America for national and international markets. We seek to help create a more sustainable and resilient world. With these goals in mind, we have expanded our service portfolio beyond organic to social and environmental certifications.

Visit us: https://biolatina.com

From our regional offices we serve Latin American.

Our headquaters:
Av. Javier Prado Oeste 2501, Bloom Tower Of. 802, Magdalena del Mar,
 Lima 17, Perú

EKOagros

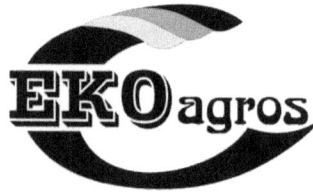

ORGANIC CERTIFICATION

Lithuania

EKOAGROS is the only institution in Lithuania for more than 20 years carrying out certification and control activities of organic production and products of national quality, also providing services of certification activities in accordance with the foreign national and private standards in foreign countries. From year 2017 EKOAGROS is accredited as certifying agent to conduct certification activities on crops, wild crops, livestock and handling operations in accordance with USDA NOP.

Contact information:
EKOAGROS
Address K. Donelaicio str. 33, LT-44240 Kaunas, Lithuania
Tel. No. +370 37 20 31 81
Website: www.ekoagros.lt

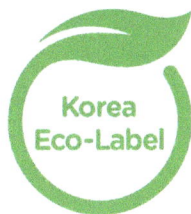

Korea
Eco-Label

Republic of Korea

The Korea Eco-labelling is a certification system enforced by the Ministry of Environment and KEITI(Korea Environmental Industry & Technology Institute). Since its foundation in April 1992, the system has certified a wide range of eco-friendly products, which were selected as excellent not only in terms of their environmental-friendliness, but also for their quality and performance during their life cycle. Korea Eco-labelling is voluntary certification scheme to attach logo to products with superior environmental quality throughout their lifecycle to other products of the same use, and thus to provide product information to consumers. For 30 years, the scheme has launched plenty of eco-labelling product standards covering personal and household goods, construction materials, office equipment furniture, etc. It products categories which cover all aspects of products, such as reduction of use of harmful substances, energy saving, resource saving, etc. As of April 30th 2021, 169 criterias(=standards), and certifications for 18,250 products(4,549 companies) have maintained.

Contact:
Korea Environmental Industry & Technology Institute(KEITI)
Office of Korea Eco-Label Innovation
Address: 215, Jinheung-ro, Eunpyeong-gu, Seoul, Repulic of Korea
T: +82 2 2284 1518
F: +82 2 2284 1526
E: accolly@keiti.re.kr
W: www.keiti.re.kr

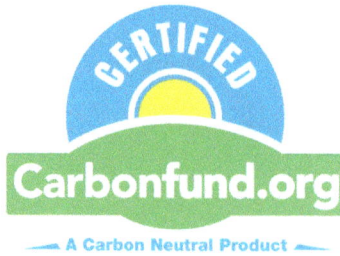

USA

The Carbonfree® Product Certification is a meaningful, transparent way for you to provide environmentally-responsible, carbon neutral products to your customers. By determining a product's carbon footprint, reducing it where possible and offsetting remaining emissions through our third-party validated carbon reduction projects, companies can:

- Differentiate their brand and product
- Increase sales and market share
- Improve customer loyalty
- Strengthen corporate social responsibility & environmental goals

The Carbonfree® Product Certification Program is proud to be part of Amazon's Climate Pledge Friendly Program!
Carbonfund.org is leading the fight against climate change, making it easy and affordable to reduce & offset climate impact and hasten the transition to a clean energy future.

Contact:

O: 240.247.0630 ext 633
C: 203.257.7808
M: 853 Main Street, East Aurora, NY, 14052

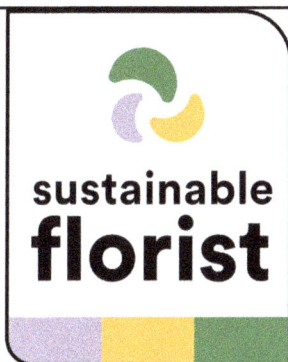

Netherland

For more than 25 years, the independent Dutch foundation SMK works from professional knowledge with companies to improve the sustainability of products and business management. SMK cooperates with an extensive stakeholder network of governments, producers, branch and non-governmental organisations, retailers, consultancies, researchers. The SMK Boards of Experts establish objective criteria for more sustainable products and services. SMK's transparent work processes, third party audits and certifications are conducted according to international certification standards, mostly under supervision of the Dutch Accreditation Council. Besides, SMK is Competent Body of the EU Ecolabel. SMK keeps an extensive database of sustainability criteria.

Contact:
Bezuidenhoutseweg 105 - 2594 AC Den Haag
Telefoon: 070-3586300
Mobiel: 06-82311031
(niet op woensdag)
www.smk.nl

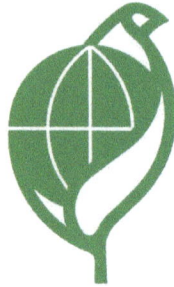

Taiwan

The Green Mark GM) Program was launched by the Environmental Protection Administration of Taiwan (TEPA) in 1992. As the official Type I eco-labeling program, it is in compliance with the requirements of the international stadard, ISO 14024 and is considered an important tool to promote green consumption and production .

To improve the GM application/review mechanism and introduce a third party certification scheme, TEPA promulgated the «Guideline for the Management of Certification Organizations for Environmental Protection Products" in June 2012. Both Environment and Development Foundation (EDF) and the Taiwan Testing and Certification Center (ETC) were commissioned by TEPA as official certifiers. With the expansion of certification capacity and authorization of the certification decision, the certification time was greatly reduced.

Contact :

Website: www.edf.org.tw
TEL: 886-3-5910008 #39
E-mail: lhliu@edf.org.tw

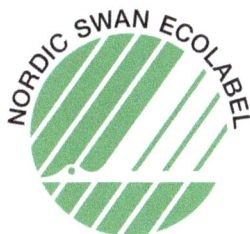

Denmark, Finland, Norway, Iceland, Sweden

The Nordic Swan Ecolabel
The Nordic Swan Ecolabel is the official Nordic ecolabel supported by all Nordic Governments. It is among the world›s strictest and most recognised environmental certifications.

The Nordic Swan Ecolabel is a Type I environmental labelling program established in 1989 by the Nordic Council of Ministers, connect¬ing policy, people, and businesses with the mission to make it easy to make the environmentally best choice. Nordic Ecolabelling is the non-profit organisation responsible for the Nordic Swan Ecolabel.

The organisation offers independent third-party certification and support for a wide range of product areas and services, ensuring that they comply with the Nordic Swan Ecolabel's strict requirements through documentation and inspections.

30 years of experience and expertise has made the Nordic Swan Ecolabel a powerful tool that paves the way to a sustainable future by giving producers a recipe on how to develop more environmentally sustainable products, and giving consumers credible guidance by helping them identify products that are among the environmentally best.

Globally, you can find more than 25,000 Nordic Swan ecolabelled products. 93% of all Nordic consumers recognise the Nordic Swan Ecolabel as a brand, and 74% believe that the Nordic Swan Ecolabel makes it easier for them to make envi¬ronmentally friendly choices (IPSOS 2019).

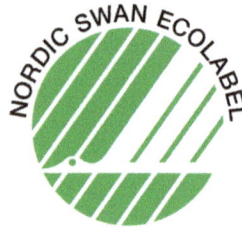

Denmark, Finland, Norway, Iceland, Sweden

Securing a sustainable future
The Nordic Swan Ecolabel works to reduce the overall environmental impact from production and consumption and contributes significantly to UN Sustainable Development Goal 12: Responsible consumption and production.

To ensure maximum environmental impact, the Nordic Swan Ecolabel sets product specific requirements and evaluates the environmental impact of a product in all relevant stages of a product lifecycle - from raw materials, production, and use, to waste, re-use and recycling.

Common to all products certified with the Nordic Swan Ecolabel is that they meet strict environmental and health requirements. All requirements must be documented and are verified by Nordic Ecolabelling. Nordic Ecolabelling regularly reviews and tightens the requirements.

Therefore, certifications are time-limited and companies must re-apply to ensure sustainable development.

International website:
Nordic-ecolabel.org
National websites:
Denmark: ecolabel.dk
Sweden: svanen.se
Norway: svanemerket.no   (in Norwegian)
Finland: joutsenmerkki.fi (in Finnish)
Iceland: svanurinn.is   (in Icelandic)

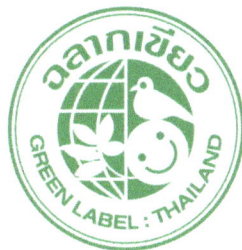

Thailand

The Thai Green Label Scheme was initiated by the Thailand Business Council for Sustainable Development (TBCSD) in October 1993. It was formally launched in August ١٩٩٤ by The Thailand Environment Institute (TEI) and Thai Industrial Standards Institute (TISI). The Green Label is an environmental certification logo awarded to specific products which have less detrimental impact on the environment in comparison with other products serving the same function. The Thai Green Label Scheme applies to all products and services, but not foods, beverage, and pharmaceuticals. Products or services which meet the Thai Green Label criteria may carry the Thai Green Label. Participation in the scheme is voluntary.

Thailand Environment Institute (TEI)
16/151 Muang Thong Thani, Bond Street,
Bangpood, Pakkred, Nonthaburi 11120 THAILAND
Tel. +66 2 503 3333 ext. 303, 315, 116
Fax. +66 2 504 4826-8
Website: http://www.tei.or.th/greenlabel/
Email: lunchakorn@tei.or.th

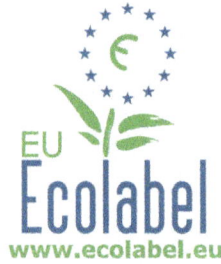

EUROPE

Established in 1992 and recognized across Europe and worldwide, the EU Eco-label is a label of environmental excellence that is awarded to products and services meeting high environmental standards throughout their life-cycle: from raw material extraction, to production, distribution and disposal. The EU Eco-label promotes the circular economy by encouraging producers to generate less waste and CO_2 during the manufacturing process. The EU Ecolabel criteria also encourages companies to develop products that are durable, easy to repair and recycle.

The EU Ecolabel criteria provide exigent guidelines for companies looking to lower their environmental impact and guarantee the efficiency of their environmental actions through third party controls. Furthermore, many companies turn to the EU Ecolabel criteria for guidance on eco-friendly best practices when developing their product lines. The EU Ecolabel helps you identify products and services that have a reduced environmental impact throughout their life cycle, from the extraction of raw material through to production, use and disposal. Recognised throughout Europe, EU Ecolabel is a voluntary label promoting environmental excellence which can be trusted.

Spain , Germany, Italy, Sweden, Greece, Portugal, Poland, Belgium, Netherlands, Estonia, Finland, Austria, Lithuania, Czech Republic, Norway, Cyprus, Ireland, Slovenia, Hungary, Romania, Croatia, Bulgaria, Malta, Slovak Republic, Latvia, Luxembourg, Iceland

Contact and more information via: http://ec.europe.eu

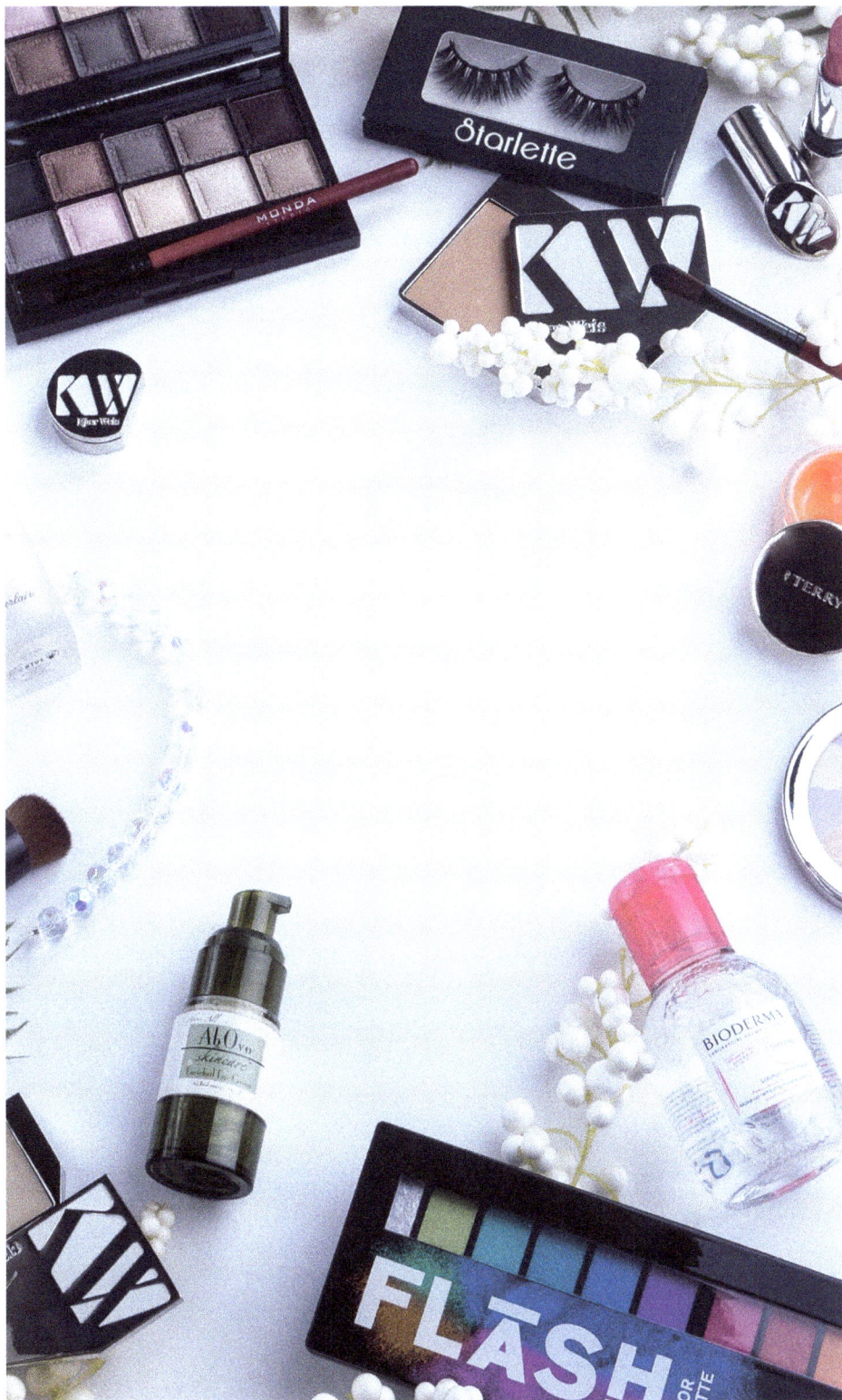

Purchasing a green cosmetic product, which is influenced by the preference and purchase intention of the consumer, is mainly determined by the presence of eco-labels. Furthermore, the attention a consumer pays to an eco-label is also important issue in purchasing green cosmetics containing eco-labels.

By increase the amount of information about eco-labels given to consumers at the point of-purchase., the awareness of the influence of different eco-labelled goods on the environment will increase. As a consequence, additional information at the point-of-purchase will result in increased attention to an eco-label

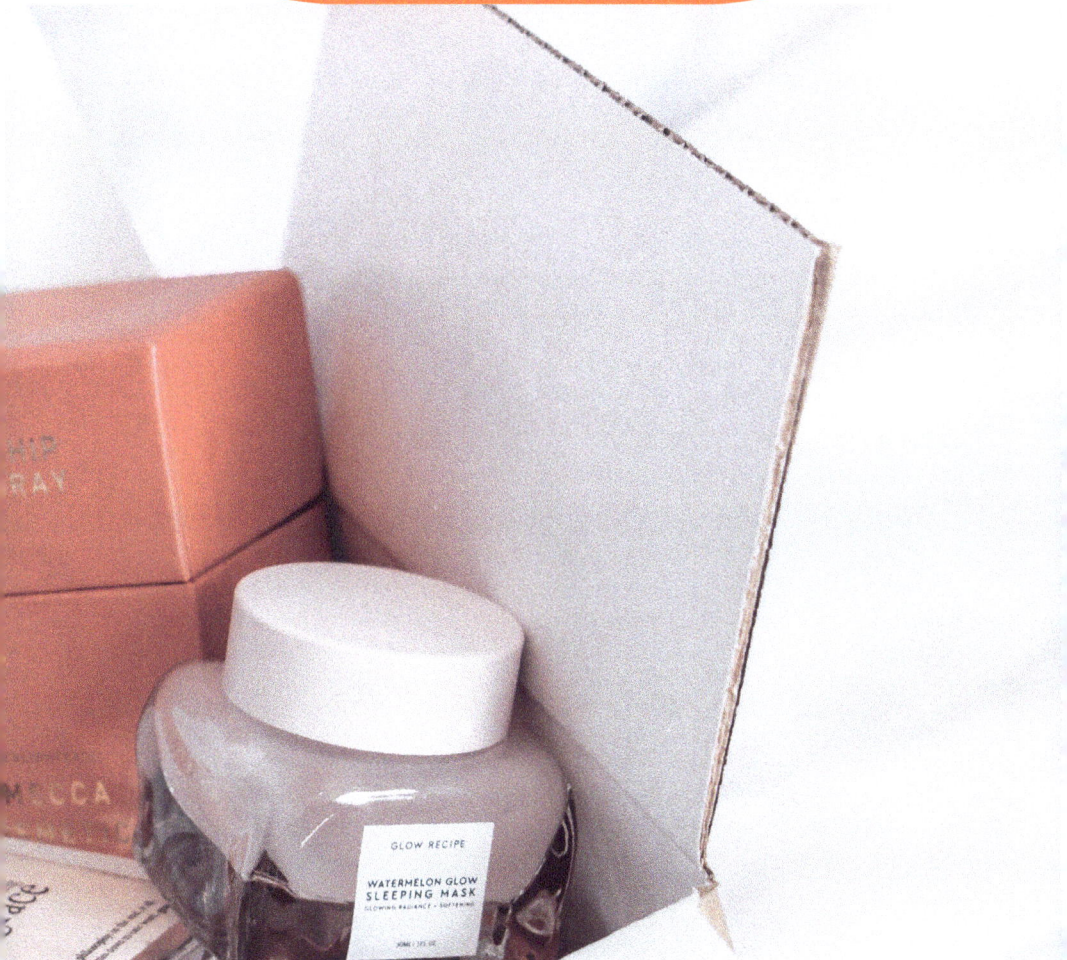

CHAPTER 5

Type II Environmental Labelling

Type II environmental labelling refers to the claims made on product labels in connection with business centers. This includes familiar claims such as recyclable, ozone-free, 60% phosphate-free, and the like. This type of labelling can be in the form of a mark or sentence on the product packaging. Some of them are valid environmental claims—and some can be completely misleading.

Usually, all countries have laws against deceptive advertisements, so why has the International Organization for Standardization discussed this issue? The answer is that it is not clear whether the environmental claims have a technical basis or whether the ad is meaningless.

Most countries have guidelines at the national level to help producers and consumers know what constitutes a true, scientifically valid claim.
There is a national standard on this in Canada. In Australia, the Consumer Commission has published guidance on this, and there are similar examples in other countries.

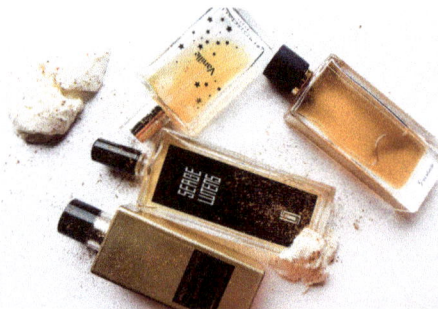

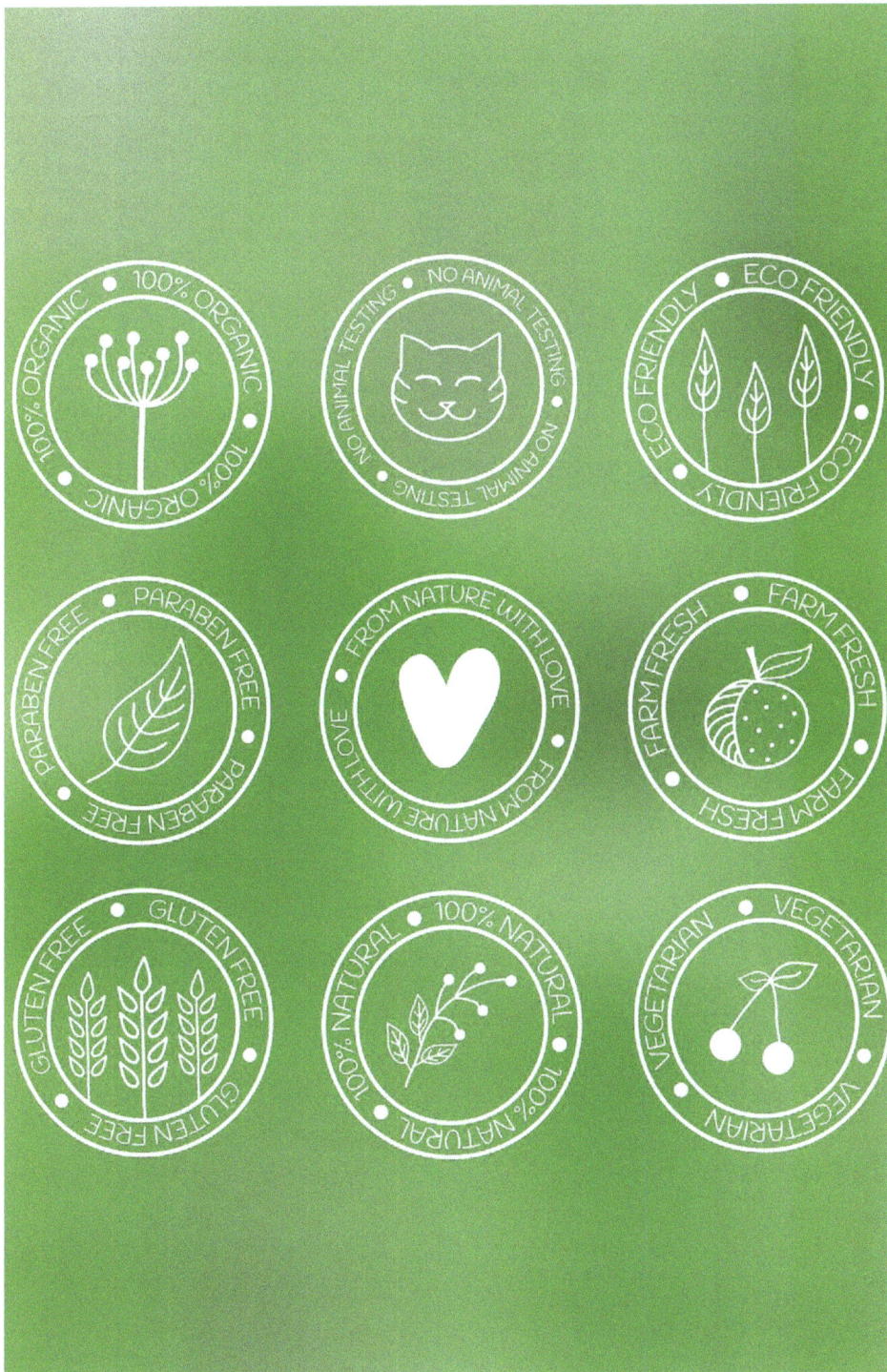

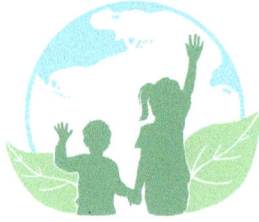

Canada

Environmental Sustain for Future kids established in Vancouver, BC Canada in 2020. (ESFK) is an international ecolabel focused on taking care of environment for future of kids.

ESFK defined as 'self-declared' environmental claims made by manufacturers and businesses based on ISO 14020 series of standards, the claimant can declare the environmental objectives and targets in relation to taking care of environment for future kids. However, this declaration will be verifiable.

Environmental Sustain for Future Kids
Vancouver, BC CANADA

Email: info@esfk.org
Web: www.esfk.org

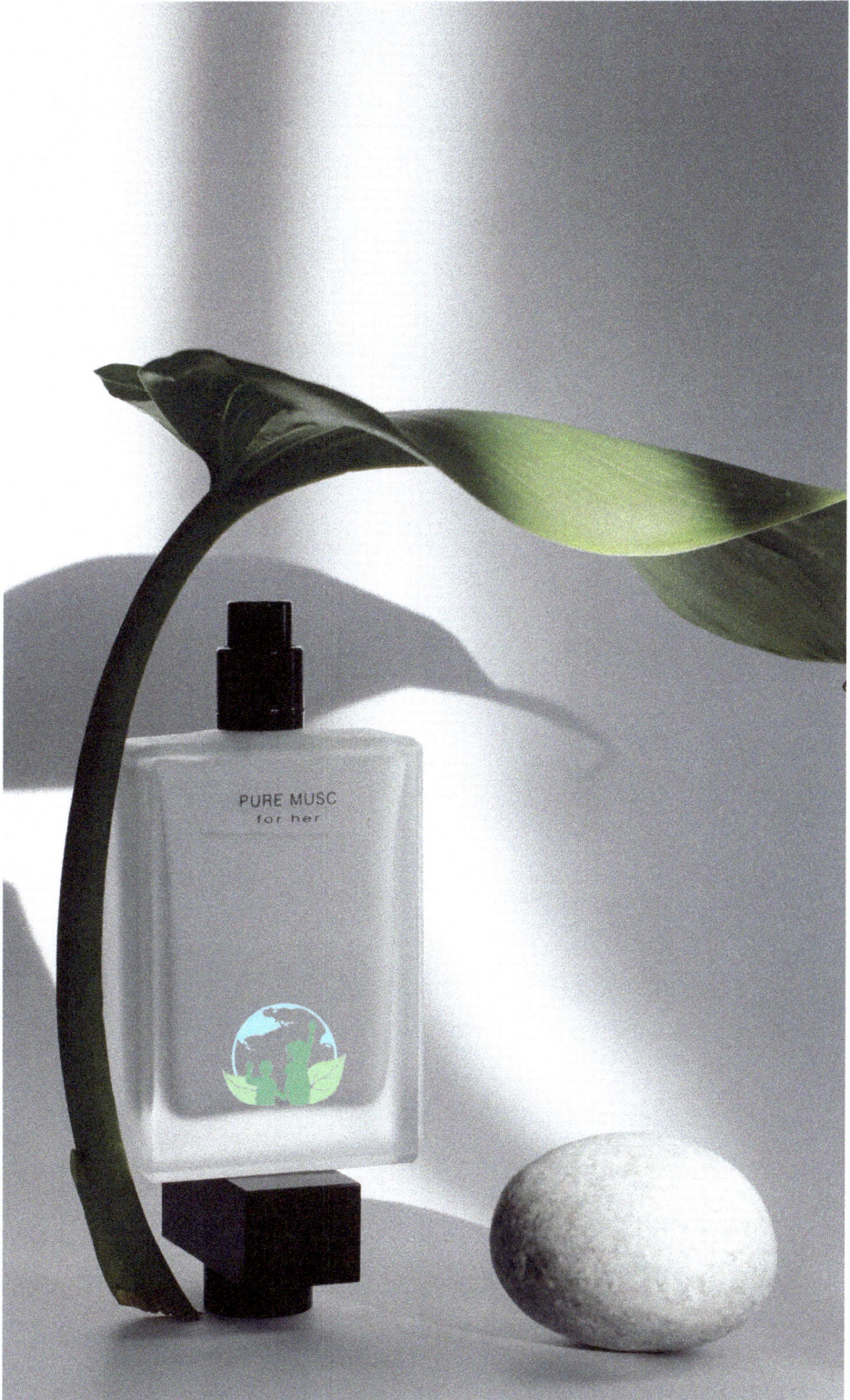

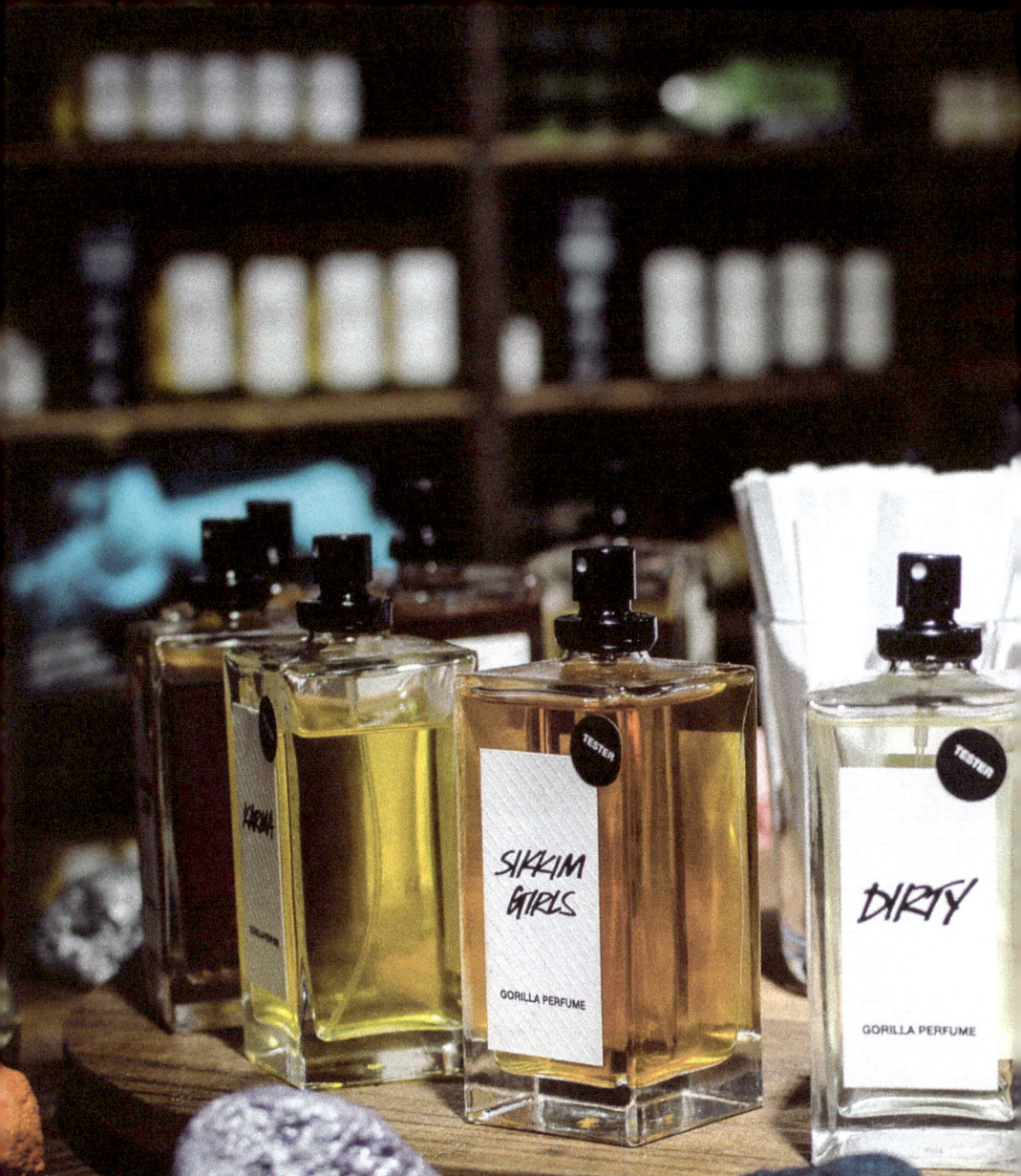

Although eco-labels are a good way to convey environmental and health information, consumers also experience some problems in understanding this visual information.

The growing number of eco-labels in green cosmetics ensures that consumers need to use different information sources in their purchase decision. Using eco-labels is an important information source in purchasing green cosmetics

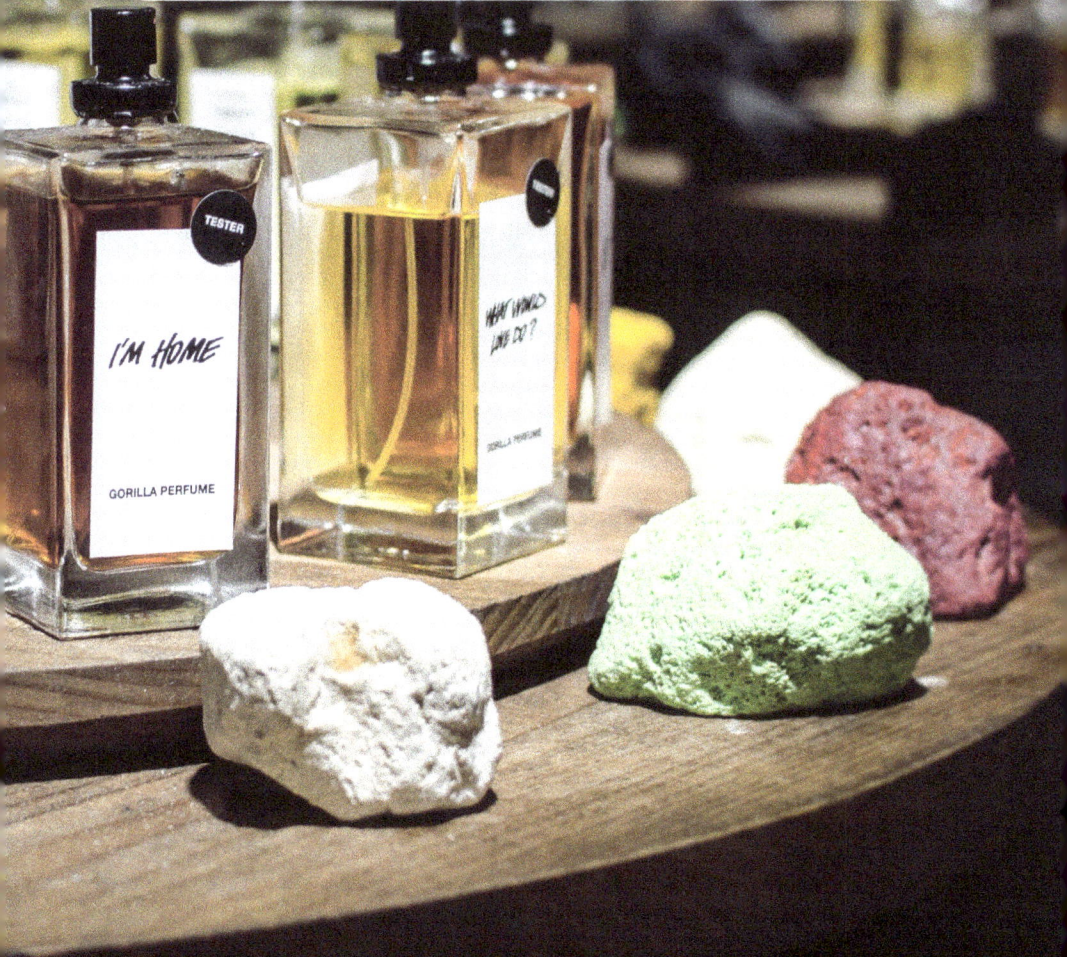

CHAPTER **6**

Type III Environmental Labelling

Type III environmental labelling is a distinct form of third-party environmental labelling pattern designed to avoid the difficulties that can result from type I labelling. Technical committee for Environment of International organization for Standardization has undertaken a new project to standardize guidelines and Type III labelling methods. One of the main objections raised by industries to Type I labelling is the basis for its management.

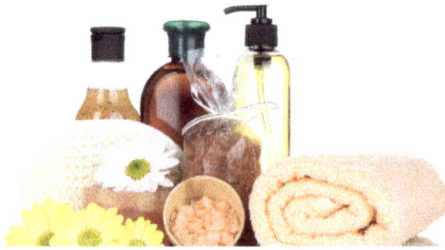

Due to the nature of the system, less than 50% of the various products on the market can meet the criteria and qualify for Type I Labelling. As long as the industry is the main supporter of other third-party models for quality systems, it is sometimes difficult for an industry to support a program that can only benefit 15% of its members. This type of labelling is currently practiced in some countries, such as Sweden, Canada, and the United States. Choosing the right product has never been easy, but Type III labelling will help because each product can have a label that describes its environmental performance and is certified by a third-party company. Consumers can then compare labels and choose their favorite products.

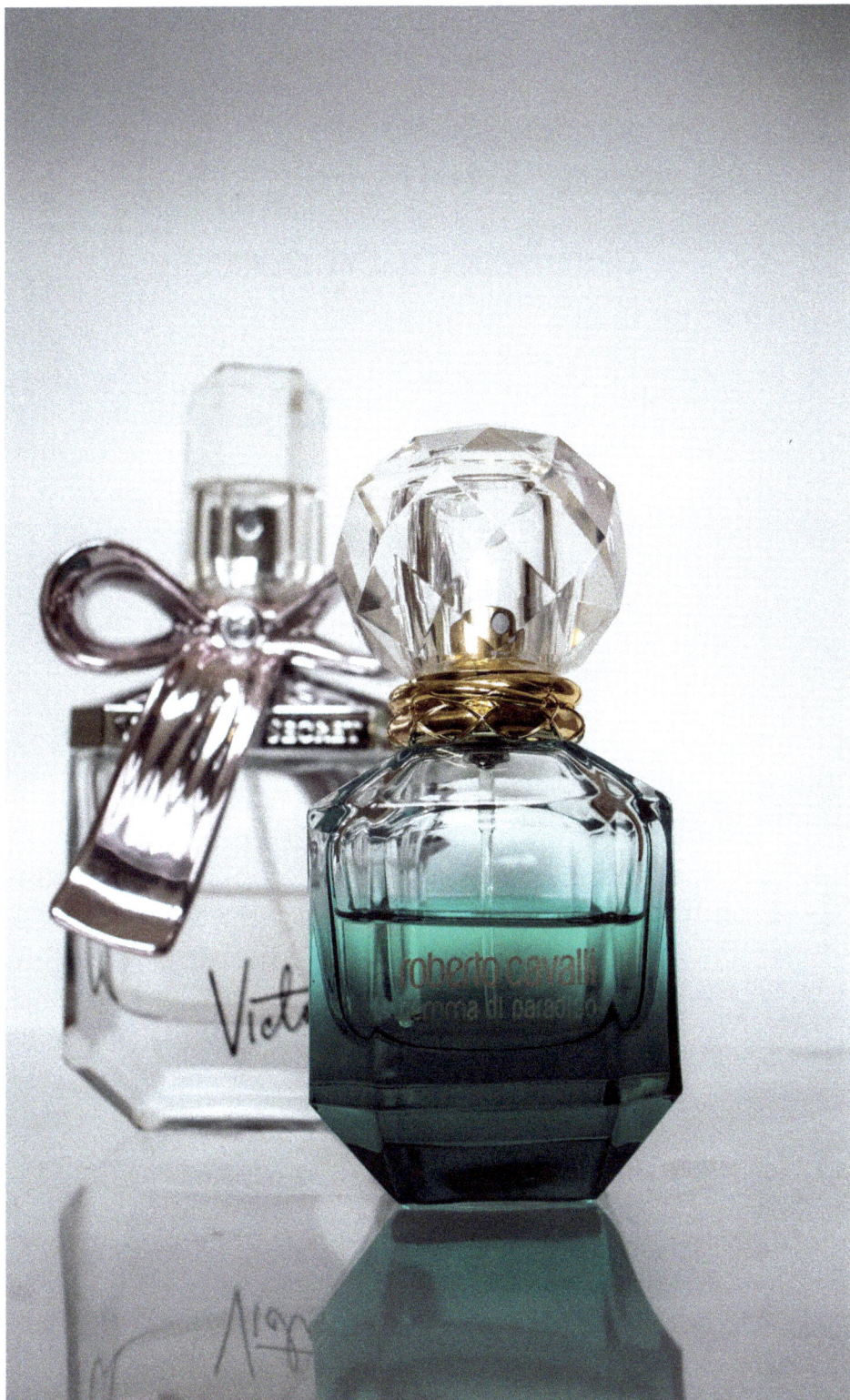

CHAPTER **7**

All about 'Eco-friendly' Health and Beauty Products

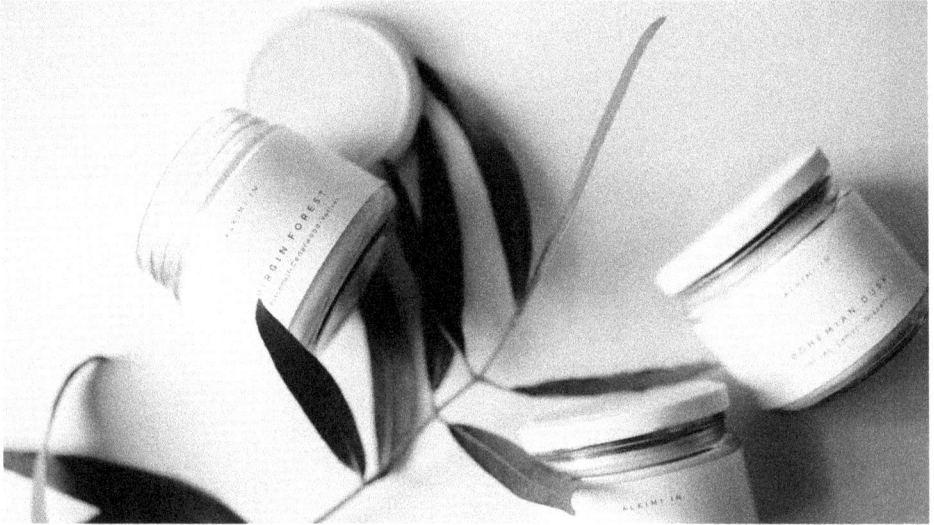

Health and beauty encompasses a variety of products, including fragrances, makeup, hair care and coloring products, sunscreen, toothpaste, and products for bathing, nail care, and shaving. The industry overlaps with other markets like chemical, health care, and petroleum.

In this book, Health and Beauty products divided into Three main catogries:

- Cosmetics
- Baby
- Hygine

Green Cosmetics:
The Push for Sustainable Beauty

As public interest in sustainability continues to climb, many cosmetic manufacturers are seeking more natural and environmentally-friendly emulsifiers and ingredients for their products. The benefits of "green" beauty products extend beyond trends — increasing studies show the toxicity of conventional cosmetics, and the natural cosmetics market continues to grow rapidly and consistently.

Manufacturing companies interested in venturing into the green market must know the details behind the sustainability movement, including the benefits of going green and the potential of the market. In modern marketing, the word "green" has become synonymous with "organic" or "healthy." When a consumer sees the phrase "green cosmetics," they will automatically make eco-friendly assumptions about the product or company.

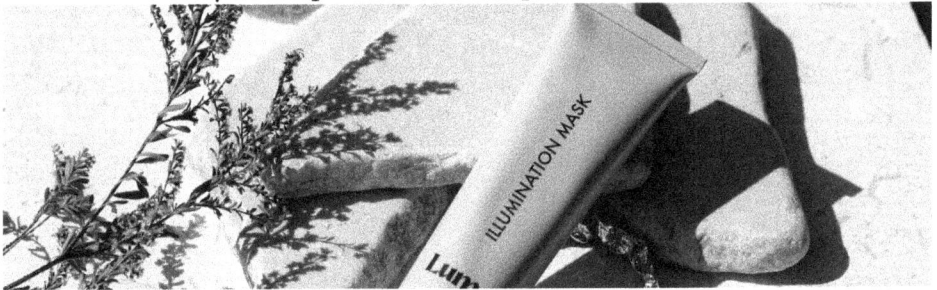

But the field of green cosmetics still needs clarification. Typically, the term is used to describe products using environmentally-friendly formulations, production practices or packaging methods. In the United States, the Federal Trade Commission (FTC) has published guidelines to clarify what green or natural means in marketing terms, though these guidelines are still loosely defined.

With respect to the cosmetics industry, "green" and "sustainable" cosmetics are defined as cosmetic products using natural ingredients produced from renewable raw materials. Many companies use petrochemical ingredients derived from petrol, a non-renewable and economically volatile resource. Bio-based oleochemicals, on the other hand, derive from renewable plant and bacteria sources and are the crux of the green cosmetics movement.

How Are Sustainable Cosmetics Made?

Cosmetics developers worldwide are doggedly pursuing these oleochemicals, along with any potential sources for them. Some examples of common sources include:

Natural Oils: Palm and coconut oils are often used to derive fatty alcohols, which are used as chemical surfactants. Other oils include argan oil and avocado oil. Glycerine, a derivative of palm oil, is a common byproduct.

Agricultural Plants: Soybeans, corn and other agricultural plants are used throughout the cosmetic industry to produce oils and alcohols. Green cosmetic emulsifiers, surfactants and biocatalysts are derived using these plants, which can be cheaply and sustainably sourced.

Bacteria: One example of a renewable resource currently under development is the Deinococcus bacteria, a bacterium studied by Deinove in France for its chemical production properties. Deinove has used the bacterium to create aromatic ingredients and pigments for the cosmetic industry, representing a potential market value in the hundreds of millions of dollars.

Manufacturers split these raw materials into oleochemicals at a processing plant. The fats or oils are divided by hydrolysis, which uses water, or alcoholysis, which uses alcohol.

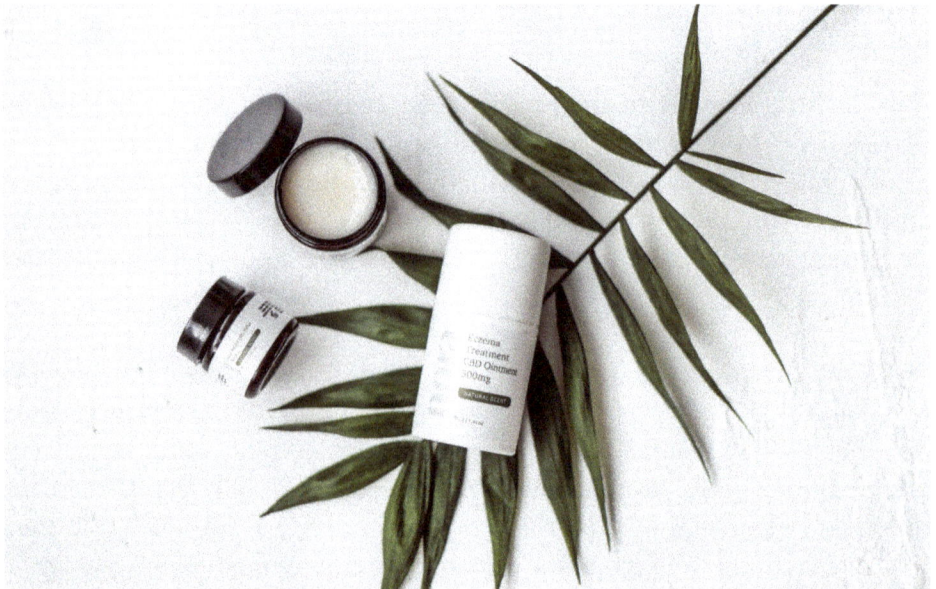

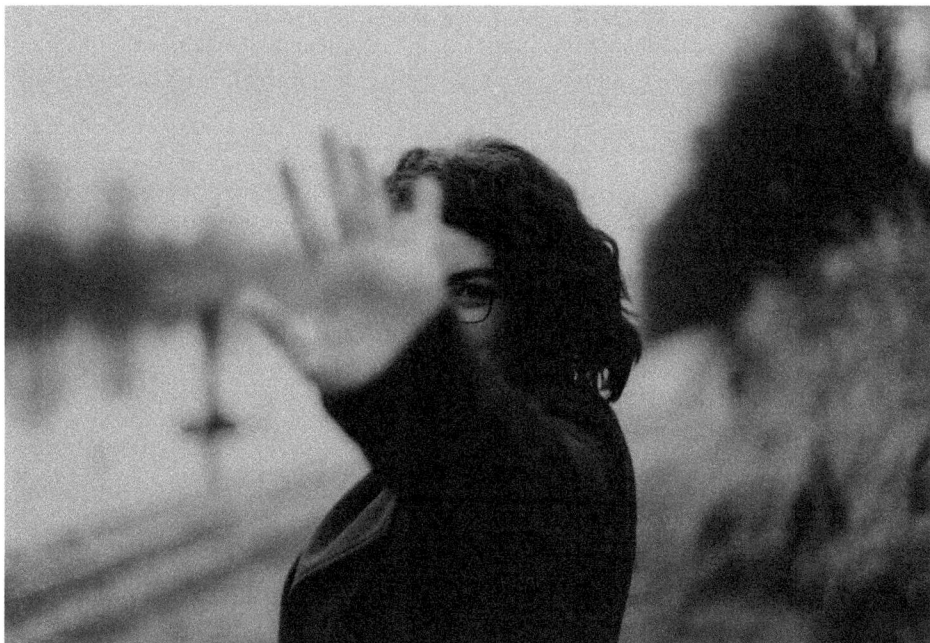

Ingredients That Aren't Sustainable

Avoid many of the toxic elements found in popular brands. These chemicals damage environmental and human health, and consumers should never read them on a "green" label.

Aluminum:

Commonly used in antiperspirants, aluminum enters the body through the underarm tissue and blocks sweat ducts. However, it has also been linked to breast cancer, Alzheimer's disease and osteoporosis.

Dibutyl phthalate (DBP):

Often found in nail products, DBP is a solvent for dyes. Considered toxic to human reproduction, it enhances the ability of other chemicals to cause genetic mutations. While Canada has banned DBP from all children's toys, no action has yet been taken against its presence in cosmetics.

Coal tar dyes:

On labels, coal tar dyes are listed as p-phenylenediamine or colors titled "CI" and followed by a five-digit number. These dyes are mixtures of petrochemicals, and they have been linked to cancer in humans.

BHA and BHT:
BHA and BHT are synthetic antioxidants used as preservatives, and they are most common in lipsticks and moisturizing creams. The European Commission has released evidence that BHA and BHT disrupt the endocrine system.

Formaldehyde-releasing preservatives:
These preservatives are present in a wide range of cosmetics, as well as in cleaning products such as toilet bowl cleaners. As their name suggests, formaldehyde-releasing preservatives continuously release small amounts of formaldehyde, a known human carcinogen.

Examples of Sustainable Cosmetics:

Many manufacturers have found success using oleochemical-based products, and beyond creating high-quality and effective products, they have gained a loyal customer following. Here are some of the most well-known, sustainable cosmetics companies and their products:

Native: Native produces deodorants with organic, natural ingredients. Native has built their brand around "simple, nontoxic ingredients you can understand." Their oleochemical-derived ingredients include shea butter, coconut oil and castor bean oil.

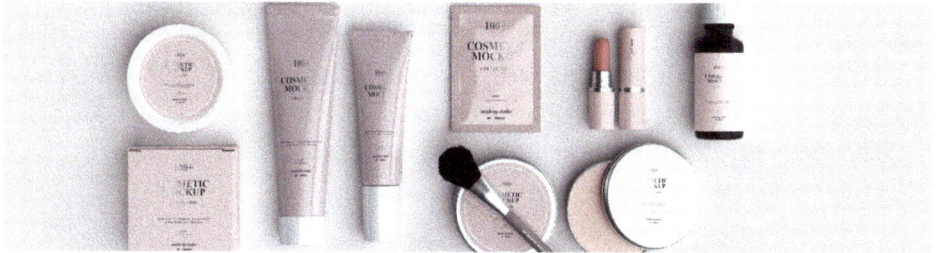

Burt's Bees: From simple beeswax candles to a lip-product empire, Burt's Bees has become an international leader in sustainability. The company creates cosmetics and personal care products, and in addition to natural, organic ingredients, it has a "no-waste" manufacturing policy. They rely on botanical oils, herbs and beeswax to come up with their world-recognized products.

RMS Beauty: RMS Beauty provides a wide range of cosmetics, from foundation to mascara. Dedicated to using organic ingredients, RMS creates non-toxic makeup products that heal and protect the skin. They use low-heat processing to ensure their ingredients remain as natural as possible.

Blissoma: Focusing on skincare, Blissoma offers a large selection of products organized by skin type and need. Their preservative-free cosmetics include natural ingredients like fruit enzymes, Vitamin C and organic herbs and grains.

Drunk Elephant: Committed to using clean, natural ingredients, Drunk Elephant manufactures a range of sustainable skin care products. They have a devoted consumer following and strive to create products that are both clinically-effective and naturally-sourced.

It's possible for any company to incorporate green materials in their cosmetics. If you want to branch into the world of sustainable, oleochemical-derived products, begin with some of these safe and effective ingredients.

Fatty Acids: Fatty acids like coconut fatty acid, stearic acid and oleic acid are green ingredients used as lubricants, adhesives and release agents, as well as emulsifiers and base stock. You can incorporate naturally derived fatty acids into a wide range of cosmetic products, including soaps, ceramic powders, lotions and creams.

Castor Oil: Made by pressing the seeds of the castor plant, castor oil is a beneficial ingredient that has a range of anti-inflammatory and pain-relieving properties. When used in hair cosmetics, materials like Jamaican Black Castor Oil both remove impurities and clarify the scalp, resulting in more effective and more eco-friendly product.

MCT Coconut Oil: Extracted from the kernel of mature coconuts, MCT Coconut oil is a highly specialized and versatile carrier oil. Light, smooth and easily absorbed into the skin, MCT oil is especially useful in skincare products. Because it doesn't leave an oily residue, MCT oil is ideal for products marketed as oil-free or for sensitive skin types.

DMDM Hydantoin: A powerful antimicrobial agent, DMDM Hydantoin is a halogen-free preservative. This eco-friendly ingredient can be added to both rinse-off and leave-on products, including eye and skin creams, shampoo and conditioner, sunscreen, liquid soap and make-up remover.

Phenoxyethanol: Inhibiting both bacteria and mold growth, phenoxyethanol is an effective preservative used in a wide range of green cosmetics, from lotions and creams to make-up and gels. Phenoxyethanol serves a variety of roles within cosmetics, including solvent, fixative and topical anesthetic functions.

Committed to sustainable manufacturing, Acme-Hardesty offers each of these green ingredients for manufacturers in the cosmetics industry.

Why Buy Natural and Sustainable Cosmetics

Environmental Responsibility

Modern consumers have a growing global consciousness, and they care about social and environmental responsibility. One of the main benefits of sustainable products is their kinder environmental impact.

Every week, new stories surface about dangerous carbon outputs or vast plastic floats in the ocean. Many petrochemicals in conventional cosmetics are toxic pollutants and degrade the environment as well as our bodies. As we become more ecologically aware, consumers demand natural, low-polluting products.

A recent example of pollution and consumer demand is the ban of microbeads. Microbeads are tiny pieces of plastic found in many shower scrubs and exfoliating products. However, they do not dissolve, and in 2015, a study reported that over eight trillion microbeads were being washed into our waterways every day. Later that year, U.S. President Barack Obama signed a bill banning the small plastics, illustrating that environmental stewardship is an increasing priority to the nation and its consumers.

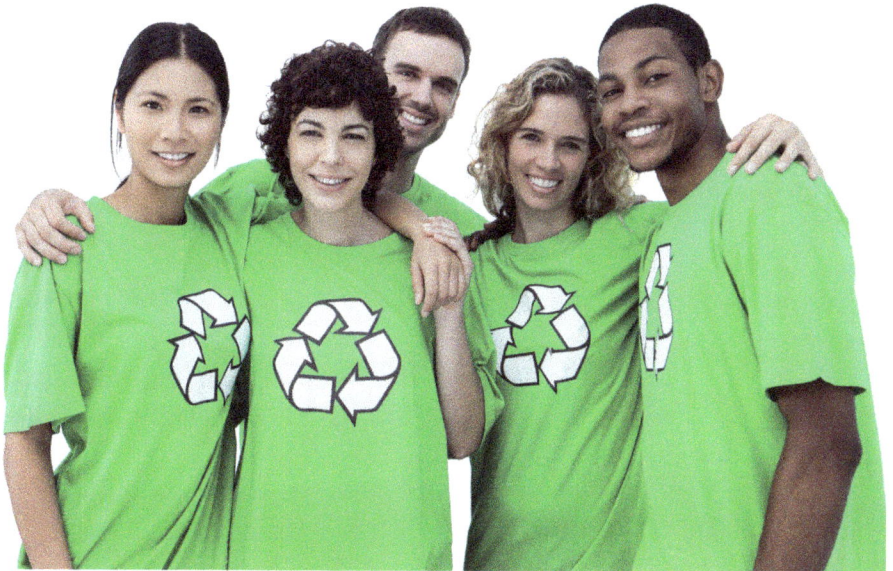

Increased Effectiveness
Natural and oleochemical ingredients are less likely to cause skin irritation or allergic reactions. Without synthetic, toxic chemicals or artificial colors, sustainable products rely on the healing properties found naturally in plants and animals — the ingredients humans have been using for centuries. Consider glycerine, a natural derivative of palm oil. The clear, non-toxic liquid is used in soaps, pharmaceuticals and cosmetics. Since it is a humectant, glycerine can retain water, making it an excellent moisturizer. Glycerine enhances the body's hygroscopic characteristics, encouraging the skin to absorb and hold on to water. As a non-irritating substance, it can be applied anywhere on the body. It is an effective anti-aging ingredient and, due to its anti-microbial properties, can also serve as an acne treatment.

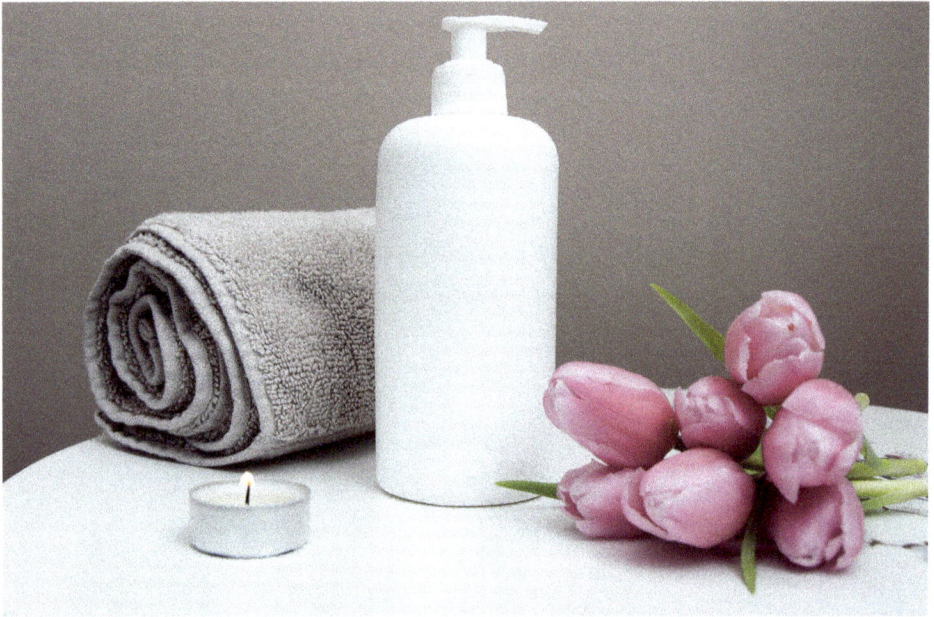

Long-Term Health
While petrochemicals may deliver short-term results, the long-term effects can be highly toxic to humans and the environment. Years of synthetic cosmetics use has been traced to headaches, eye damage, acne, hormonal imbalance and premature aging. Phthalates have even been linked to cancer and type II diabetes. By choosing sustainable cosmetics, a consumer forgoes the stress and uncertainty of toxic, synthetic products and invests in their long-term health and beauty.

Why Produce Green Cosmetics?

1. Improved Product Quality

High-quality cosmetics provide effective results without putting the consumer at risk. However, many petrochemical products, like mineral oil, present a low level of toxicity to users. When aerosolized and inhaled, such products have been shown to be allergens and, as some studies suggest, may cause cancer. With most bio-based products, the toxicity to the end-user is reduced, creating safer, higher-quality products.

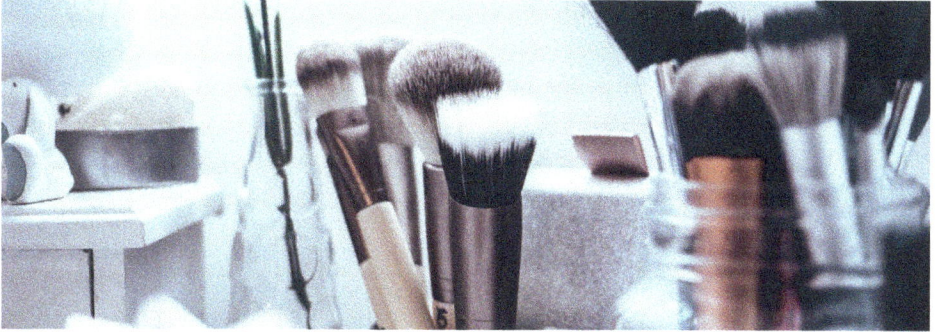

2. Enhances Brand Reputation

Green products send a message to consumers — this company is committed to quality, safety and sustainability, and is worthy of your trust. As more and more people grow concerned about synthetic products, consumers are looking for companies that practice transparency and honesty. By moving towards sustainable, green products, you show your global and social awareness. This promotes customer loyalty to a brand, not just to products. People will begin — and continue — to purchase a company's products because they agree with its mission.

3. Increases Corporate Responsibility

Green cosmetics also present a unique opportunity for cosmetics manufacturers to focus on corporate responsibility. In addition to the positive impacts green marketing can have on a company's image, taking the extra steps of sustainable sourcing or packaging can also make a significant impact. When a company increases its sustainability initiatives, it takes ownership for its impact on global health and economies. By taking corporate responsibility for its manufacturing, a business gains authority and respect among consumers as well as suppliers and other members of the distribution chain.

The Future of Sustainable Cosmetics

Manufacturers shifting to sustainable cosmetics production have a promising future. The growing interest in sustainable cosmetics has had a significant effect on the cosmetics market. With an increasing number of consumers and retailers demanding cosmetics with natural or sustainable ingredients, the green cosmetics market has experienced a 15 percent annual growth rate.

This growth rate far outpaces that global personal care and cosmetics industry, which is currently sustaining an overall 5 percent annual growth rate. By 2025, the organic beauty market will reach $25.11 billion. Within the personal care industry, the oleochemicals market is increasing as cosmetic manufacturers continue to turn away from petrochemicals. Fatty acids, in particular, should experience boosts on the green side of the market, considering that they accounted for 57 percent of the total oleochemical product demand in 2013.

The Asia-Pacific region is an area of particular interest for this market since the region accounted for 41.9 percent of the total oleochemicals market in 2013 for its abundance of raw materials and large consumer base. Both figures are unsurprising considering the quantities of bulk cosmetic glycerine regularly exported from the region. As petrochemicals continue to experience volatility in the market, turning to sustainable material sources may be the best long-term decision for cosmetics manufacturers worldwide.

Consumers are increasingly demanding sustainable products that are not toxic to themselves or the environment. The natural market is growing exponentially, and choosing raw, natural materials will cement your brand as a safe choice — both environmentally and economically.

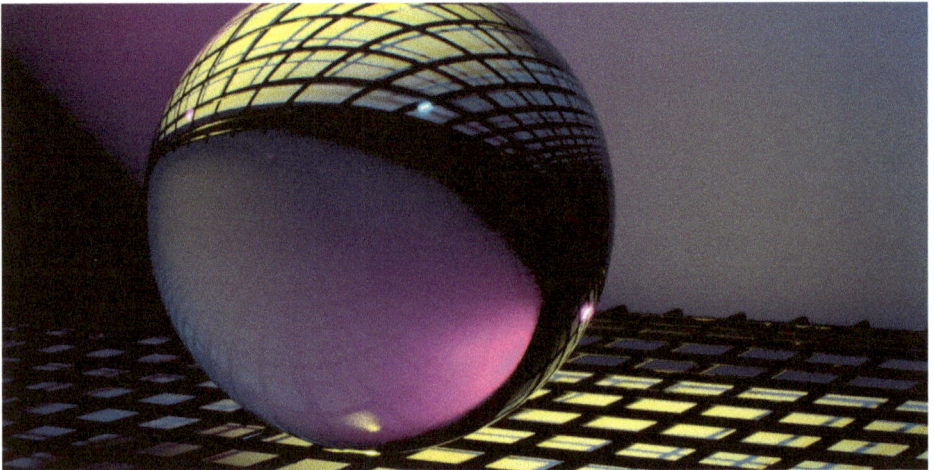

EU and UK Cosmetic product definition:

Based on the definition of the cosmetic products, products that may seem to be cosmetics, like nail wraps, a comb or a toothbrush, therefore aren't cosmetics, even though they are placed in contact with the external parts of the human body, and their primary function is to change appearance, but they wouldn't be considered a substance or a mixture.

A cosmetic product in Europe and UK is defined in the Regulation 1223/2009 as follows:

'cosmetic product' means any substance or mixture intended to be placed in contact with the external parts of the human body (epidermis, hair system, nails, lips and external genital organs) or with the teeth and the mucous membranes of the oral cavity with a view exclusively or mainly to cleaning them, perfuming them, changing their appearance, protecting them, keeping them in good condition or correcting body odours. (EU Regulation 1223/2009, Article 2.1.a)

Since products have to be placed in contact with the external parts of the human body or with the teeth and the mucous membranes of the oral cavity, any product intended to be ingested, inhaled, injected or implanted into the human body would also not be considered a cosmetic product in the EU or the UK. Breast implants then aren't cosmetics, even though their primary function is also to change appearance.

The product has to be a:

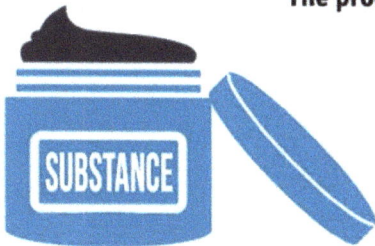

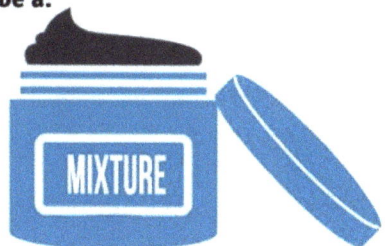

SUBSTANCE

MIXTURE

CLASSES OF COSMETIC PRODUCTS:

Cosmetic product may include:

creams, emulsions, lotions, gels and oils for the skin,
face masks,
tinted bases (liquids, pastes, powders),
make-up powders,
after-bath powders,
hygienic powders,
toilet soaps,
deodorant soaps,
perfumes, toilet waters and eau de Cologne,
bath and shower preparations (salts, foams, oils, gels),
depilatories,
deodorants and antiperspirants,
hair colorants,
products for waving, straightening and fixing hair,
hair-setting products,
hair-cleansing products (lotions, powders, shampoos),
hair-conditioning products (lotions, creams, oils),
hairdressing products (lotions, lacquers, brilliantines),
shaving products (creams, foams, lotions),
make-up and products removing make-up,
products intended for application to the lips,
products for care of the teeth and the mouth,
products for nail care and make-up,
products for external intimate hygiene,
sunbathing products,
products for tanning without sun,
skin-whitening products,
anti-wrinkle products

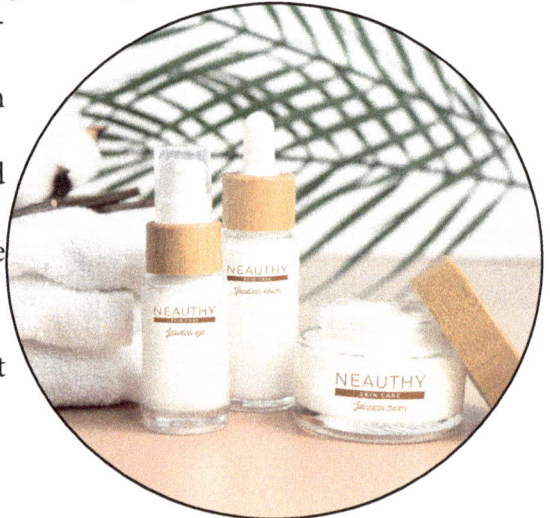

The Cosmetic Product has to be intended to place in contact with:

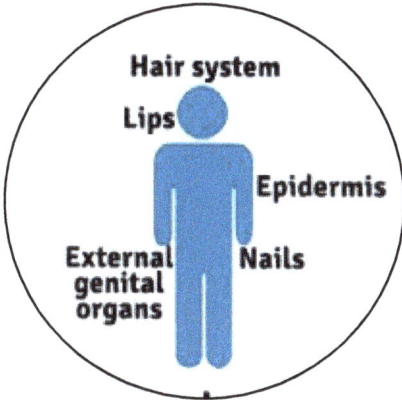

External Parts of the human body

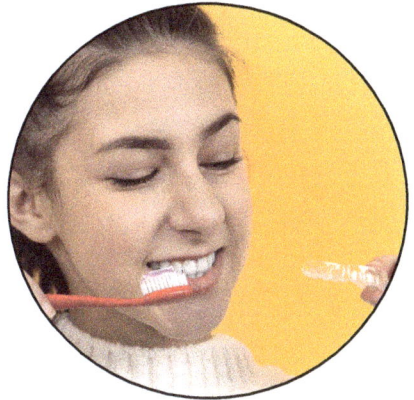

Teeth

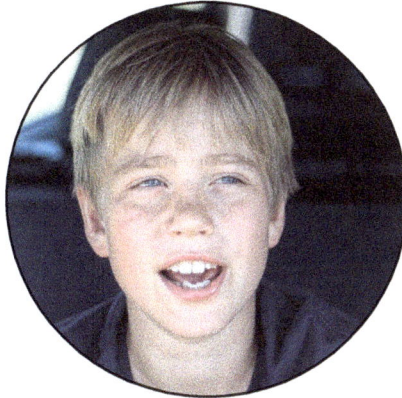

Mucous membranes of the oral cavity

The assessment of whether a product is a ECO friendly cosmetic product has to be made on the basis of a case-by-case assessment, taking into account all characteristics of the products.

The purpose of cosmetic product has to be exclusively or mainly:

The prod

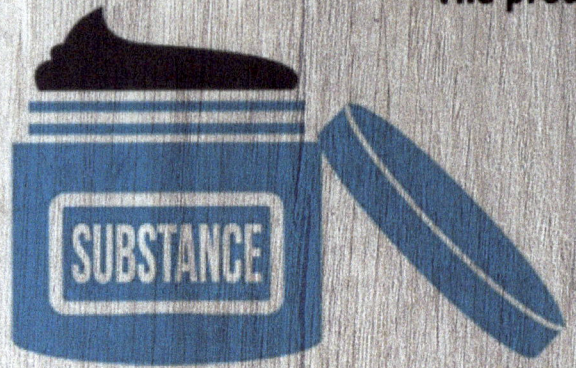

SUBSTANCE

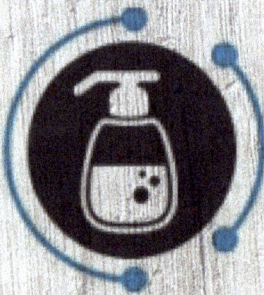

Clean

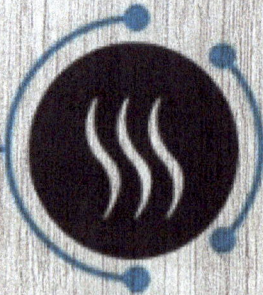

Correct body odours

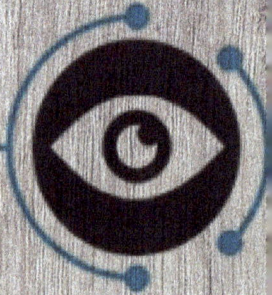

Change appearance

...us to be a:

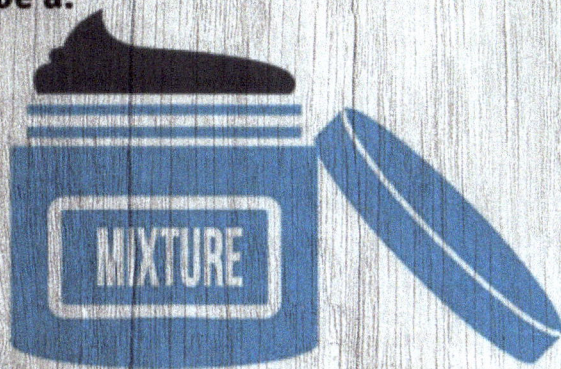

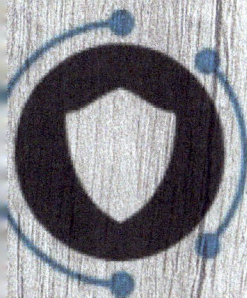

Protect

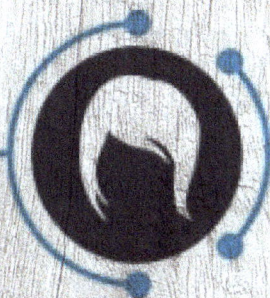

Keep in good condition

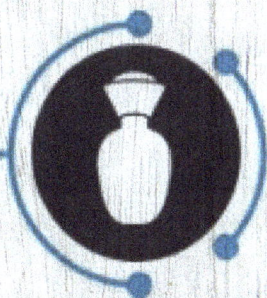

Perfume

Cosmetics FAQs:
What is meant by vegan cosmetics?
When a beauty product is marked as vegan, it means the same thing a vegan diet does. This label infers that the product does not contain any animal or its byproducts in it.

What is the difference between vegan makeup and regular makeup?
Most often, the difference between vegan and vegetarian cosmetics is that products labeled "vegetarian" will contain natural animal-made ingredients, most commonly beeswax and honey, which are avoided by vegans. Many green beauty brands that aren't 100% vegan will state that they're vegetarian. ... Testing Ingredients.

What is cruelty free in cosmetics?
Cruelty-free cosmetics is a category containing all cosmetics that have not been tested on animals. ... Many companies brand themselves as cruelty-free but still use raw materials that have been tested on animals.

"Cruelty-free" can be used to imply that:

- Neither the product nor its ingredients have ever been tested on animals. This is highly unlikely however, as almost all ingredients in use today have been tested on animals somewhere, at some time, by someone — and could be tested again.
- While the ingredients have been tested on animals, the final product has not.
- The manufacturer itself did not conduct animal tests but instead relied on a supplier to test for them — or relied on another company's previous animal-test results.
- Either the ingredients or the product have not been tested on animals within the last five, ten, or twenty years (but perhaps were before, and could be again).
- As in the case of the CCIC's Leaping Bunny Program, neither the ingredients nor the products have been tested on animals after a certification date and will not be tested on animals in the future.

Can skin care products cause allergic reaction?

Personal care products like makeup, skin cream, and fragrances also commonly cause rashes. It's not well understood how chemical compounds in personal care products trigger these rashes, called allergic contact dermatitis.

Can you suddenly become allergic to something?

Allergies can develop at any point in a person's life. Usually, allergies first appear early in life and become a lifelong issue. However, allergies can start unexpectedly as an adult. A family history of allergies puts you at a higher risk of developing allergies some time in your life.

How to Prevent Cosmetic Allergies?

Avoid ingredients in cosmetics and skincare products that are irritating to your skin. Look for labels such as "hypoallergenic", "sensitivity tested", "paraben-free", "phthalate-free", "non-comedogenic" and "fragrance-free".

What is a Non-GMO?

Non-GMO means a product was produced without genetic engineering and its ingredients are not derived from GMOs.

What is Paraben free?

Parabens can act like the hormone estrogen in the body and disrupt the normal function of hormone systems affecting male and female reproductive system functioning, reproductive development, fertility and birth outcomes. While nearly all beauty products use some kind of preservatives to make their products last longer, paraben-free cosmetics may be safer to use. The term "paraben-free" is meant to let consumers know that these harmful chemicals aren't a part of the product formula.

What is SLS ?

Sodium Lauryl Sulfate (SLS) strips the skin of its natural oils which causes dry skin, irritation and allergic reactions. It can also be very irritating to the eyes. Inflammatory skin reactions include itchy skin and scalp, eczema and dermatitis.

The Most Common Allergens in Health & Beauty Products;

Fragrance
Fragrance is one of the most common causes of allergic contact dermatitis in skincare products. "Fragrance can contain hundreds of components, and companies are not required to disclose all the ingredients that make up what's labeled as 'fragrance,'" he says. Fragrance-free is also not the same as unscented (unscented products might contain masking fragrances that neutralize perfume). Between the two, "fragrance-free is the better option if you have sensitive skin."

Parabens
"Parabens are a group of synthetic compounds commonly used as preservatives in a wide range of personal care products," . "They might cause an allergic reaction in certain people, and are more likely to irritate those with existing skin issues like eczema, psoriasis, and contact dermatitis."

Sulfates
Sodium laureth sulfate and sodium lauryl sulfate are two common skincare, bath, and hair product ingredients that also may cause rashes and itching.

Dyes
Dyes—most often found in hair products and more pigmented cosmetics—are another culprit; The dye ingredient which most often causes allergic reactions is paraphenylenediamine (PPD).

Benzyl Alcohol
"Benzyl alcohol is used for its fragrance, preservative abilities, and antimicrobial action, "In rare cases, it can cause a hive-like reaction."

Propylene Glycol
Propylene glycol is often used in moisturizers as a humectant to lock in moisture—and even at low concentrations, allergic reactions can occur, he warns.

Essential Oils

Last but not least? Essential oils. "They're highly concentrated substances that are extracted from various trees and plants for their fragrance and antimicrobial action," Tea tree oil is the most common essential oil allergen. Steer clear of products containing essential oils if your skin tends to be sensitive.

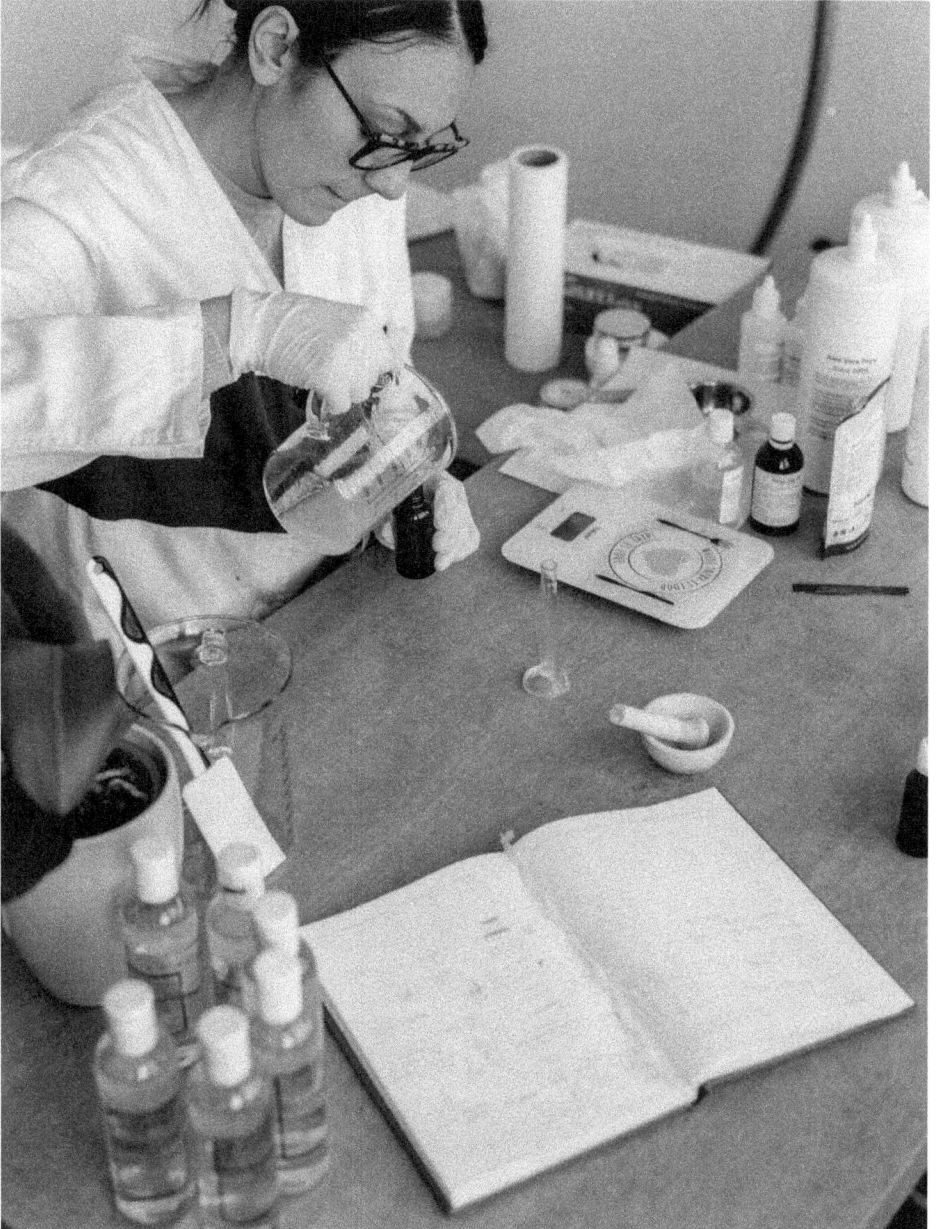

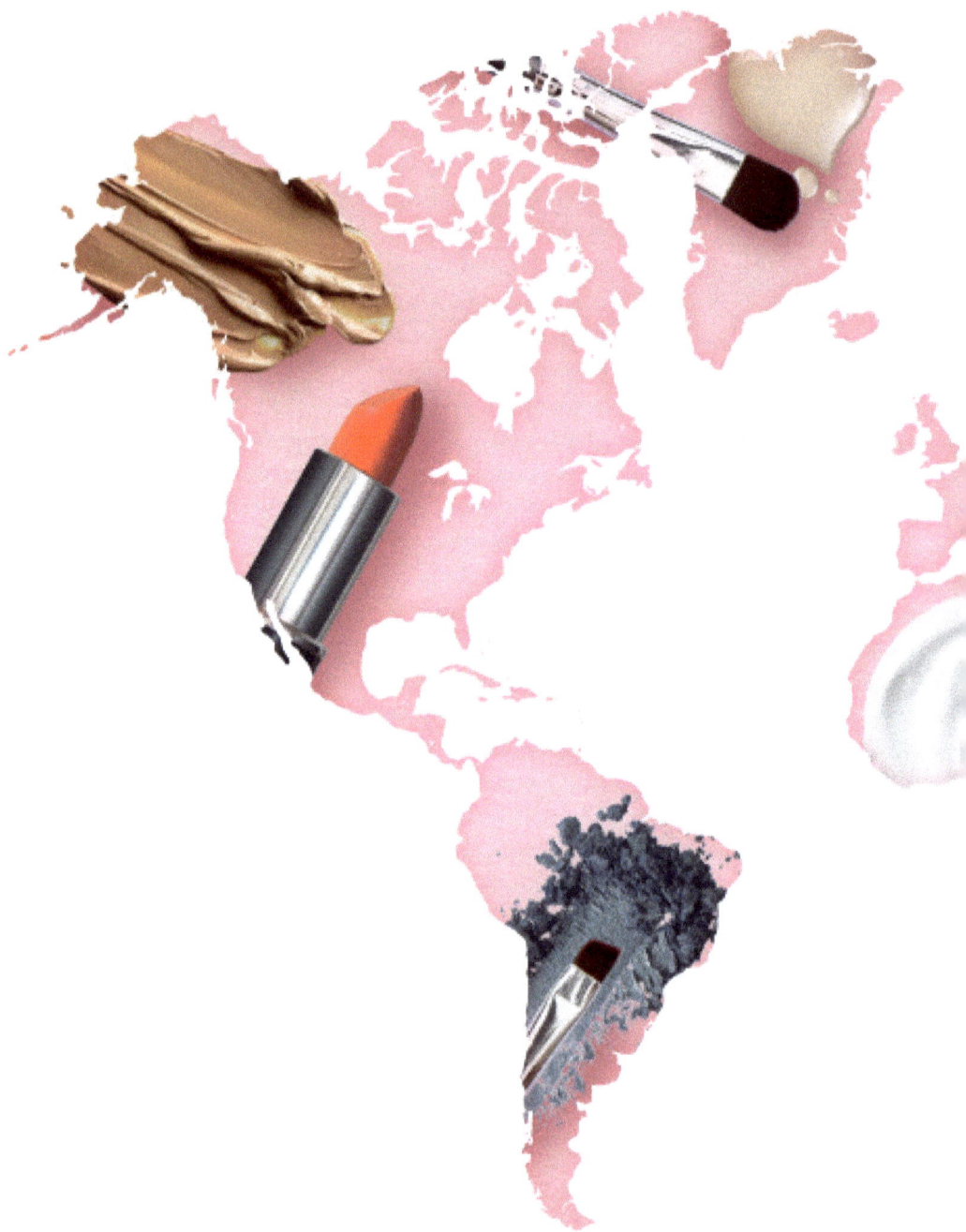

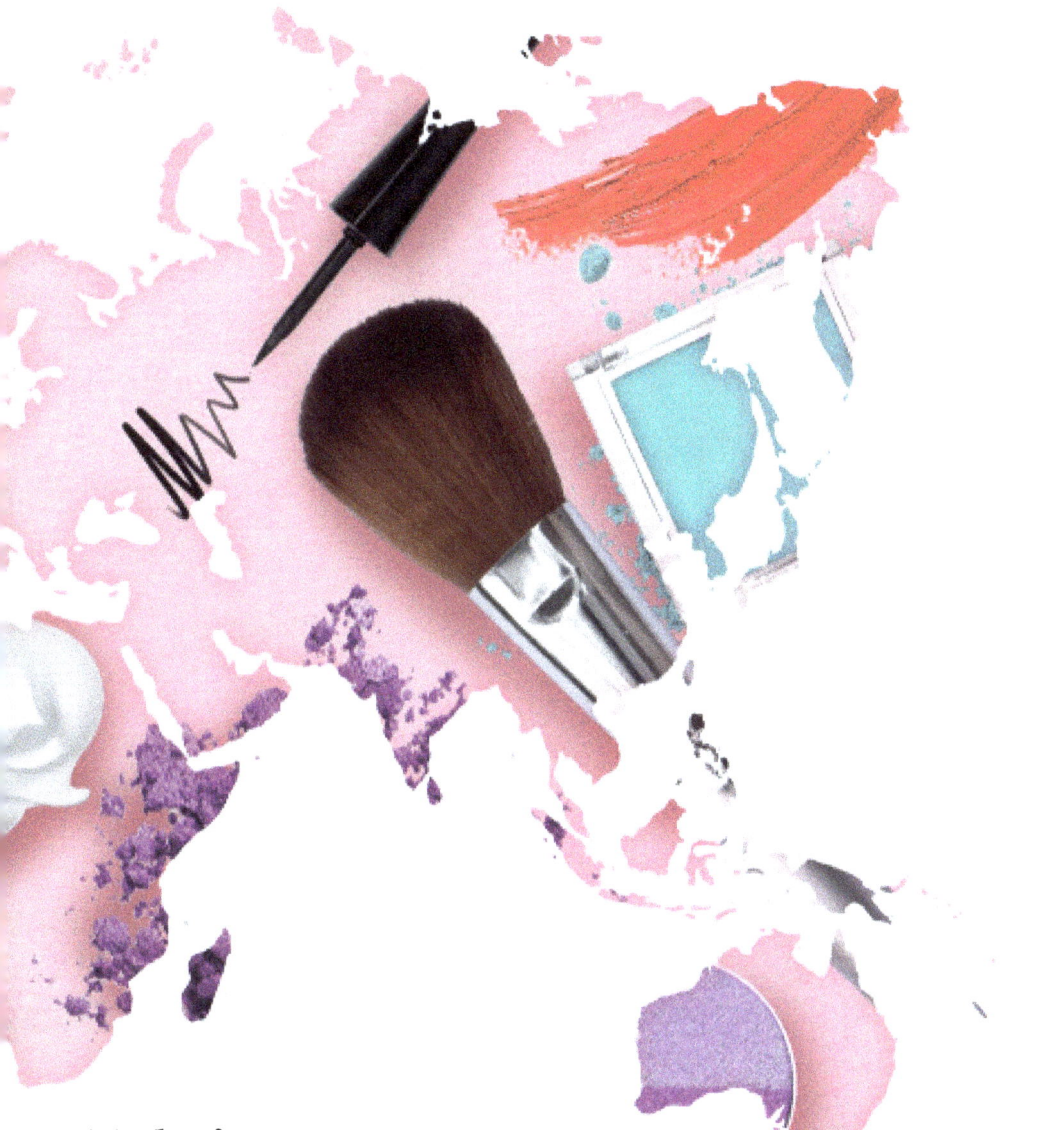

Today's sustainable paper eco friendly cosmetic packaging offers a perfect material for products that can be reduced and reused, are 100% recyclable and fully biodegradable.

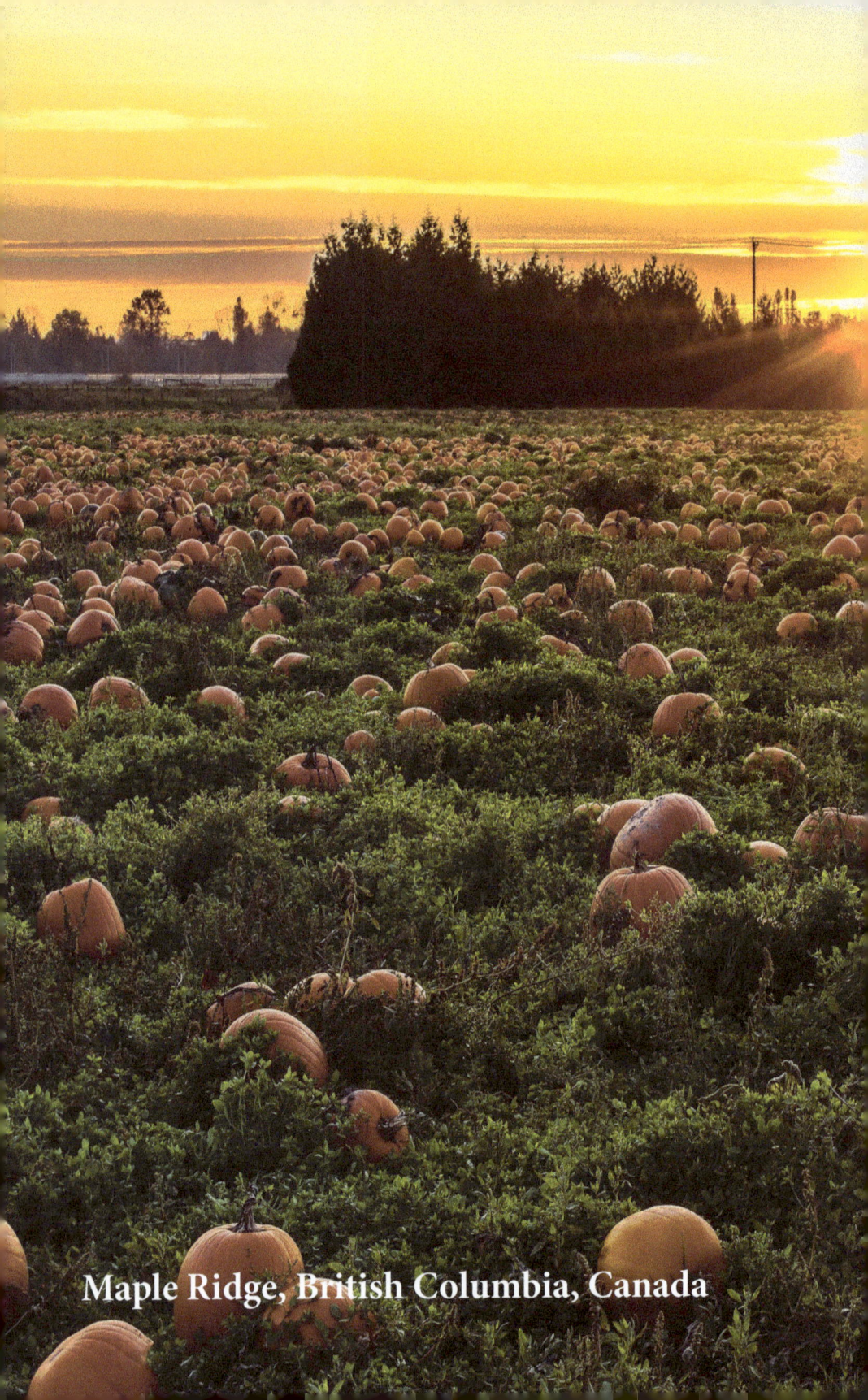

Maple Ridge, British Columbia, Canada

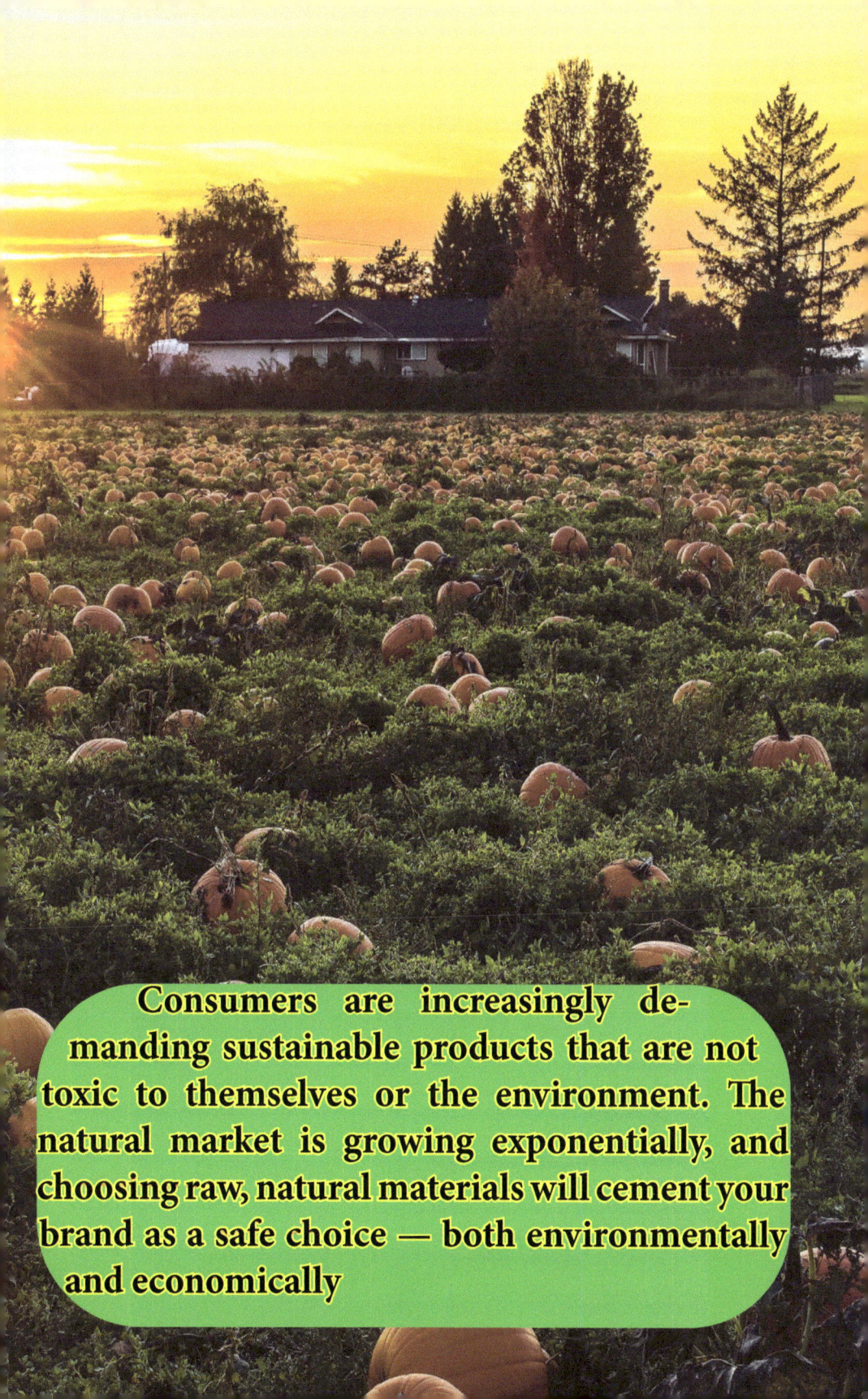

Consumers are increasingly demanding sustainable products that are not toxic to themselves or the environment. The natural market is growing exponentially, and choosing raw, natural materials will cement your brand as a safe choice — both environmentally and economically

CHAPTER **9**

Top Ten Award International Network Environmental Pioneers

T op Ten Award international Network (TTAIN) was established in 2012 to recognize outstanding individuals, groups, companies, organizations representing the best in the public works profession. TTAIN publishing books related to international Eco-labeling plans to increase public knowledge in purchasing based on the environmental impacts of products. We introduce in each volume some of the organizations that are doing their best in relation to taking care of the environmnet.

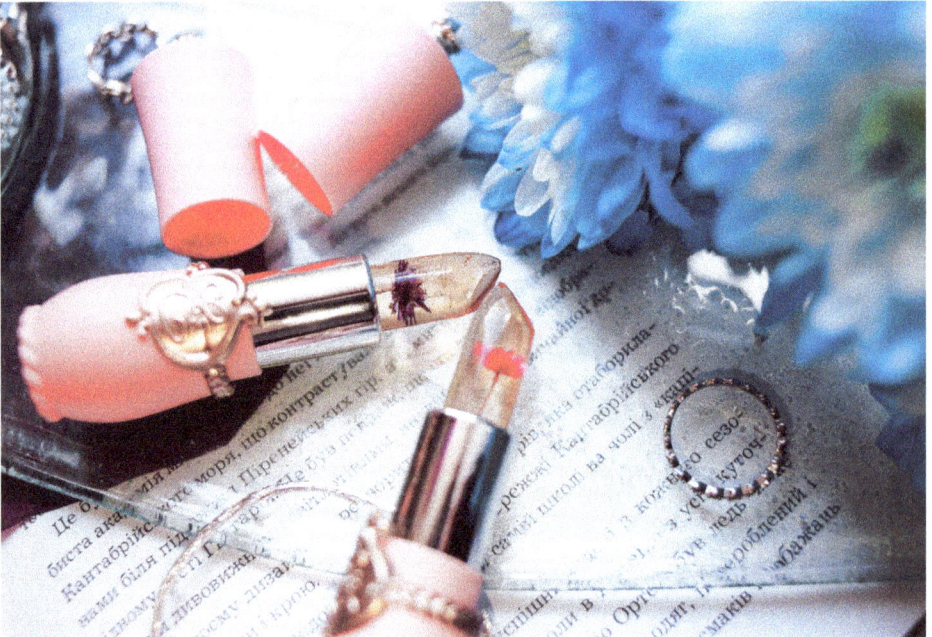

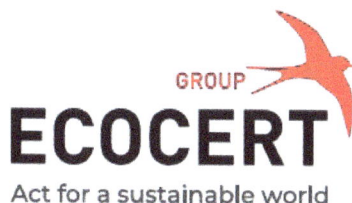

GROUP
ECOCERT
Act for a sustainable world

Canada

ECOCERT Canada, a subsidiary of the ECOCERT GROUP, has and continues to assist stakeholders in the implementation and promotion of sustainable practices through certification, consulting and training services. Committed for over 25 years to organic agriculture with Garantie Bio, ECOCERT has become the benchmark for organic certification in Canada. With more than 100 employees and its 4 offices across the country, ECOCERT Canada offers first-rate, client-focused service in both French and English to many sectors. Certification against the international COSMOS-Standard will enable you to label your product as "natural" or "organic." All the products marketed with the ECOCERT logo have been verified by our teams: from composition to processing and packaging. Consumers are thus given transparent information on the content of natural and organic ingredients that are listed on the product label.

Requirements for labeling:

Natural origin

All the ingredients are derived from natural origin except those included in a restrictive approved ingredients list (including preservatives) which are authorized in small quantities.

In general, ECOCERT certifies products as "natural" if they contain at least 95% ingredients of natural origin.

Promoting Organic

A beauty care product may be COSMOS ORGANIC certified only if:
- At least 95% of the ingredients are of natural origin,
- At least 95% of all ingredients that can be sourced as organic, must be organic
- At least 20% organic ingredients in the product (10% for rinse-off products and powders).

Contact:

Web: https://www.ecocert.com/en-CA/   Tel.: (+1) 418-838-6941

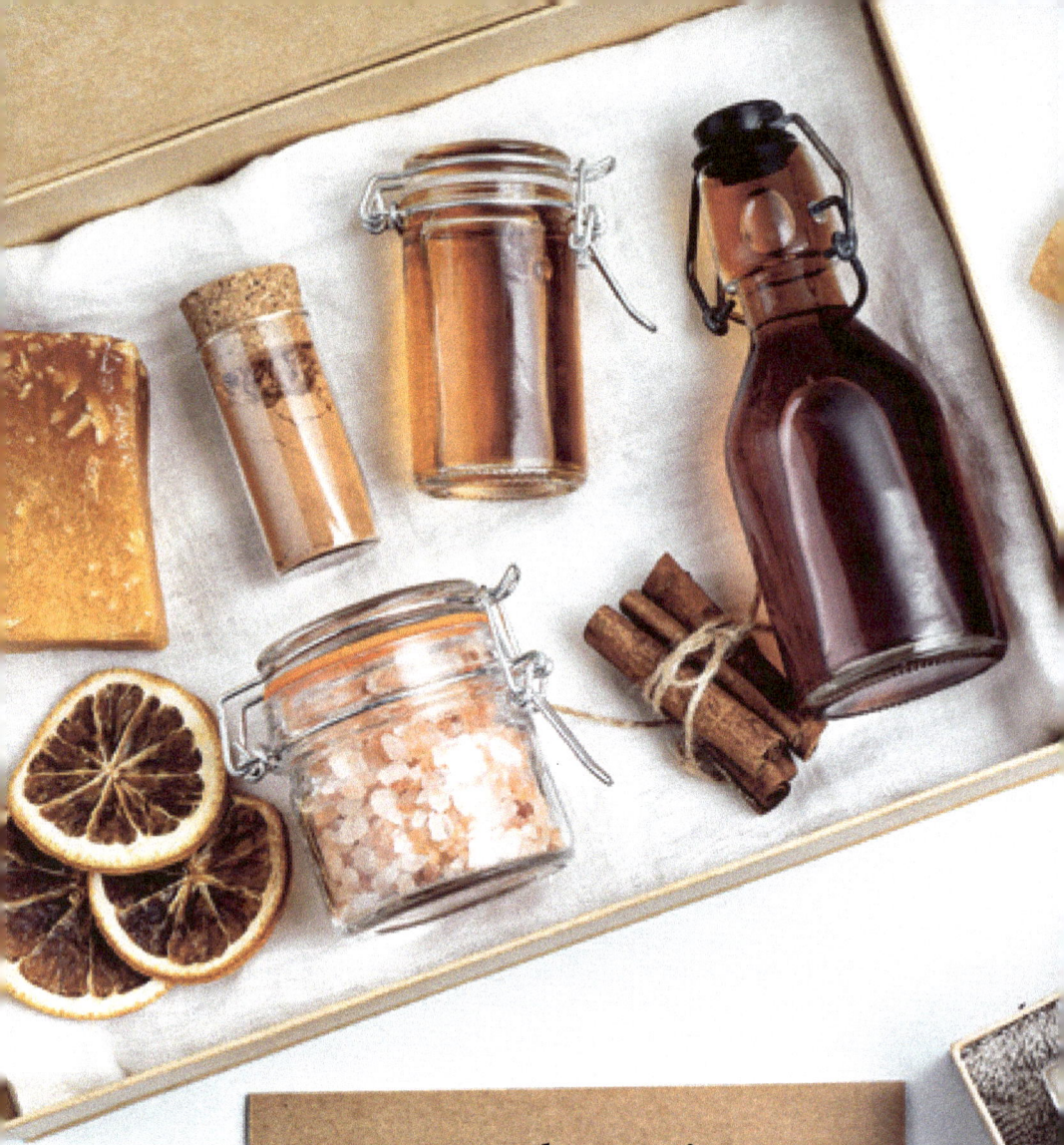

Natural cosmetics
is cosmetics which primarily contains ingredients of natural origin, processed to the minimum. In addition, natural cosmetics is expected to be ecological and ethical through the whole lifecycle of the product from the harvesting of the ingredients to the logistics.

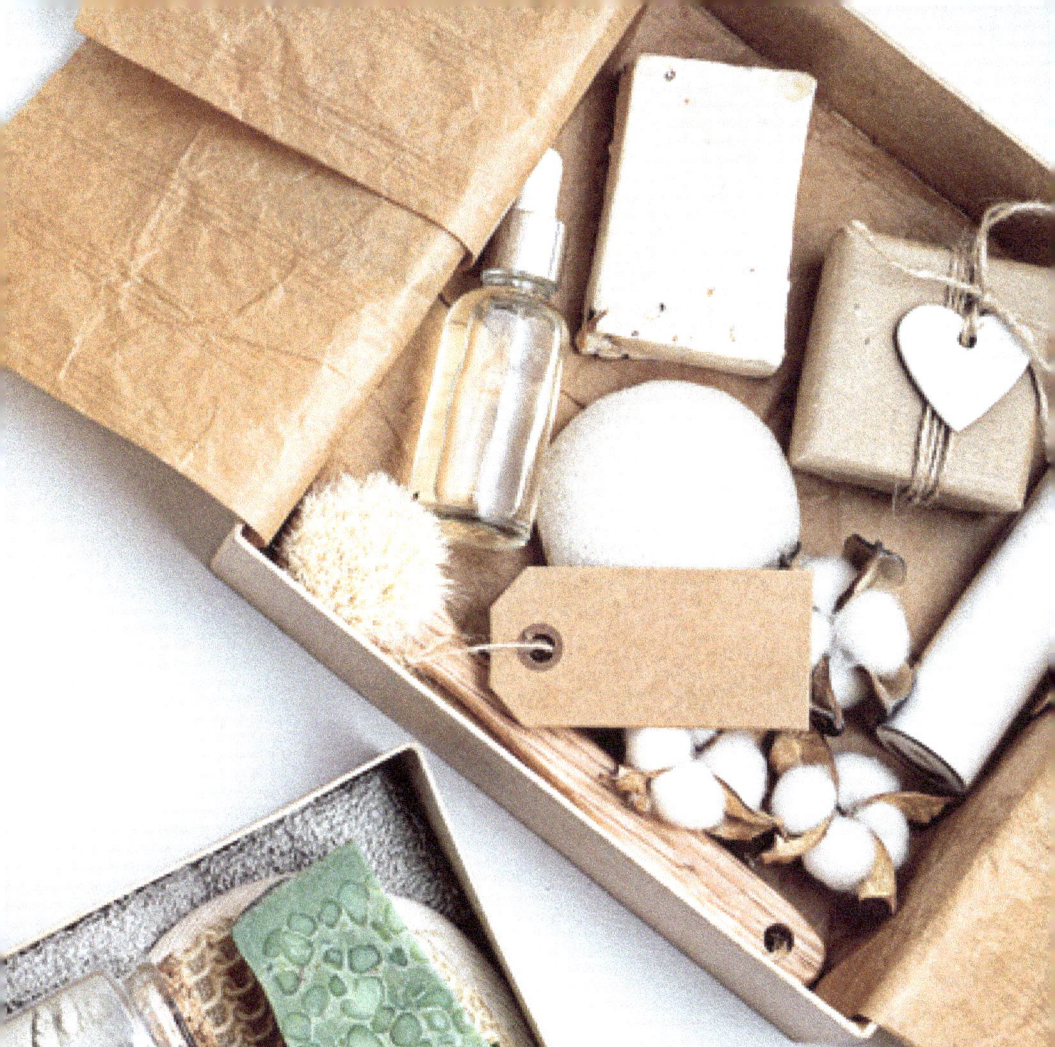

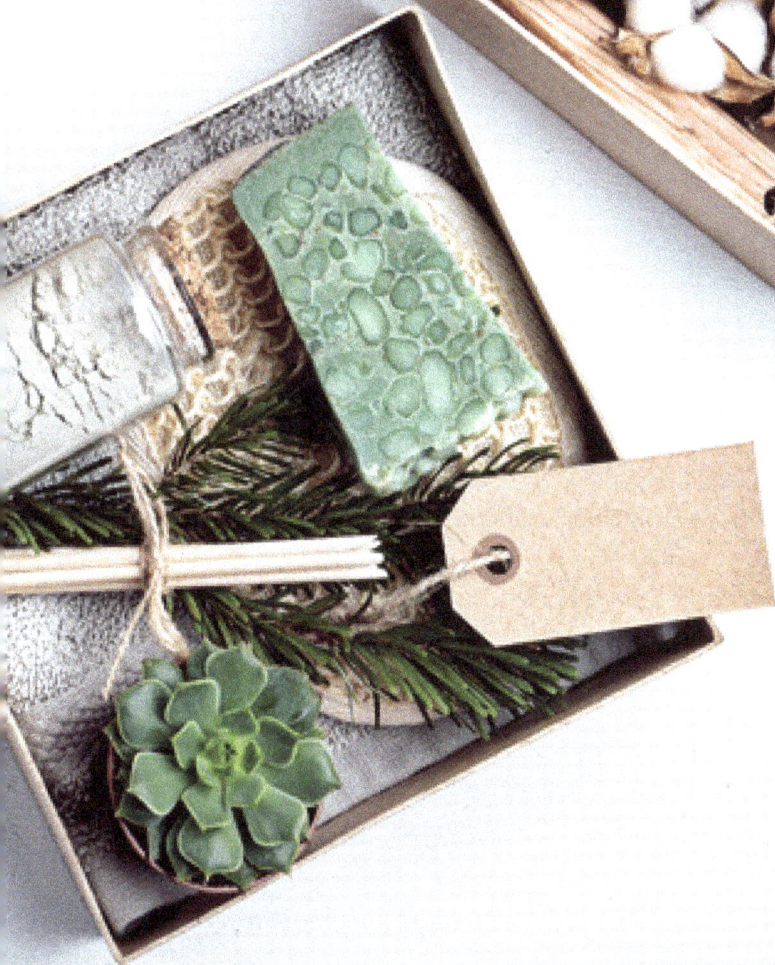

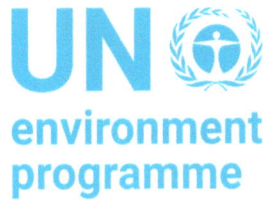

UN environment programme

UNEP

The United Nations Environment Programme (UNEP) is the leading global environmental authority that sets the global environmental agenda, promotes the coherent implementation of the environmental dimension of sustainable development within the United Nations system, and serves as an authoritative advocate for the global environment.

Our mission is to provide leadership and encourage partnership in caring for the environment by inspiring, informing, and enabling nations and peoples to improve their quality of life without compromising that of future generations.

Headquartered in Nairobi, Kenya, we work through our divisions as well as our regional, liaison and out-posted offices and a growing network of collaborating centres of excellence. We also host several environmental conventions, secretariats and inter-agency coordinating bodies. UN Environment is led by our Executive Director.

We categorize our work into seven broad thematic areas: climate change, disasters and conflicts, ecosystem management, environmental governance, chemicals and waste, resource efficiency, and environment under review. In all of our work, we maintain our overarching commitment to sustainability.

Website: www.unep.org

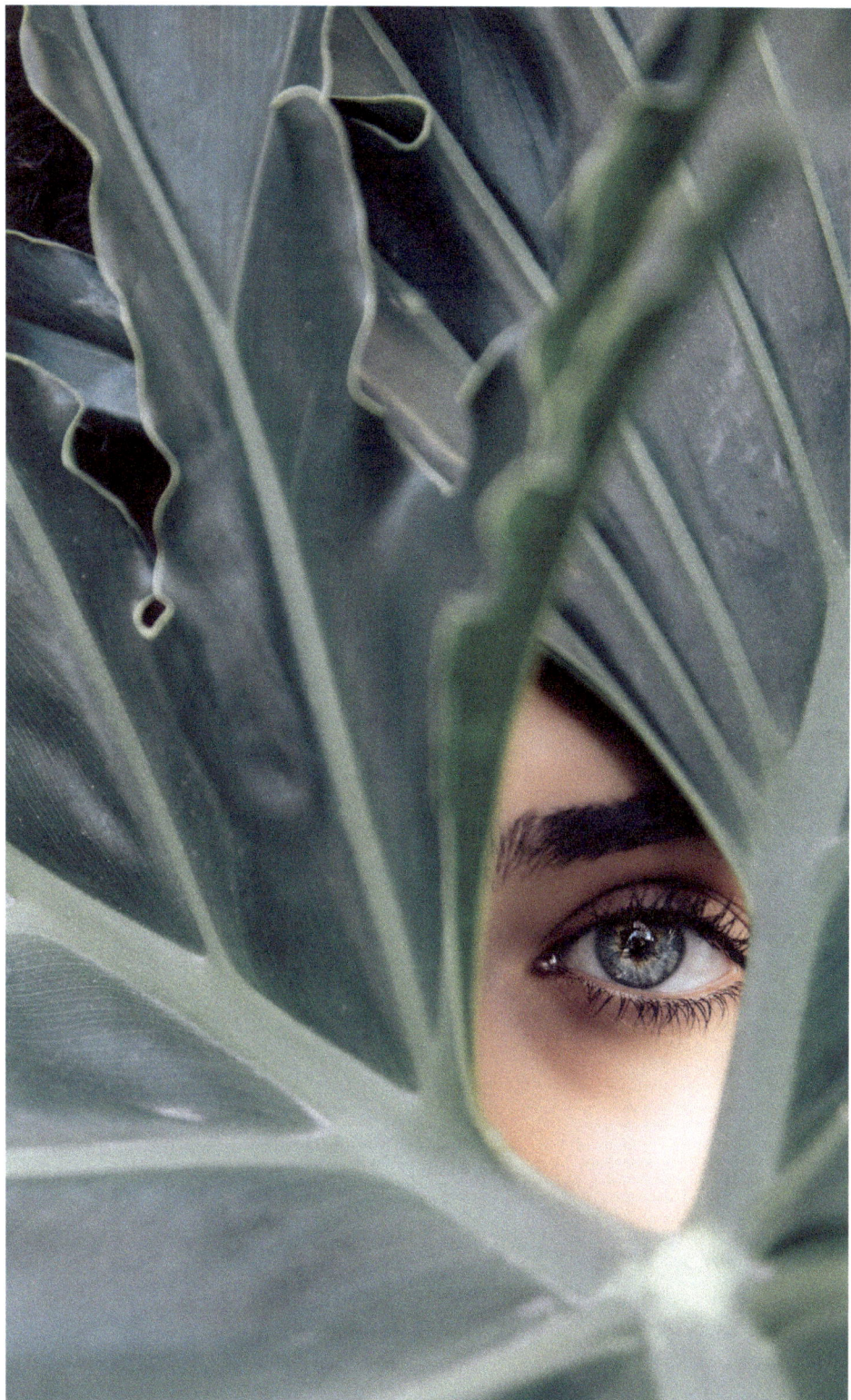

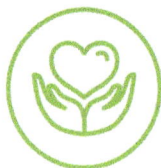

CRUELTY
FREE

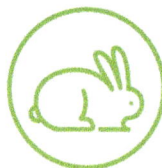

NOT TESTED
ON ANIMALS

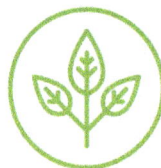

PARABEN
FREE

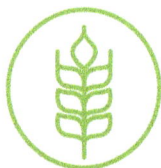

GLUTEN
FREE

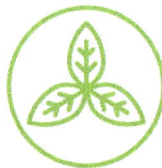

ORGANIC
PRODUCT

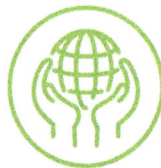

SUSTAINABLE
DEVELOPMENT

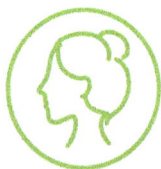

FOR ALL
SKIN TYPES

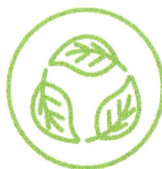

NON
TOXIC

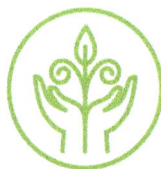

NON
GMO

Bibliography:

Amberg, N.; Magda, R. Environmental Pollution and Sustainability or the Impact of the Environmentally Conscious Measures of International Cosmetic Companies on Purchasing Organic Cosmetics. Visegrad J. Bioecon. Sustain. Dev. 2018, 1, 23.

Asadi, J., "International Environmental Labelling, Economic Consequencies, Export Magazine, July 2001

Asadi, J. 2008. Mobile Phone as management systems tools, ISO Magazine, Vol.8, No.1

Asadi, J., Eco-Labelling Standards, National Standard Magazine, Sep. 2004.

Barbieux, D.; Padula, A.D. Paths and Challenges of New Technologies: The Case of Nanotechnology-Based Cosmetics Development in Brazil. Adm. Sci. 2018, 8, 16.

Basketter, D.; Corsini, E. Can We Make Cosmetic Contact Allergy History? Cosmetics 2016, 3, 11.

Benitta Christy P & Dr. Kavitha S, "GO-GREEN TEXTILES FOR ENVIRONMENT", Advanced Engineering and Applied Sciences: An International Journal 2014; 4(3): 26-28

Chemical Week, 1999. Europe's Beef Ban Tests Precautionary Principle. (August 11).

Chaudri, S.K.; Jain, N.K. History of Cosmetics. Asian J. Pharm. 2009, 7–9, 164–167.

CHOI, J.P. Brand Extension as Informational Leverage. Review of Eco- nomic Studies, Vol. 65 (1998), pp. 655-669.

Conway, G. 2000. Genetically modified crops: risks and promise.

Corrado, M., (1989), The Greening Consumer in Britain, MORI, London

Corrado, M., (1997), Green Behaviour – Sustainable Trends, Sustainable Lives?, MORI, london, accessed via countries. Manila, Asian Development Bank 33p.

Cosmetics, Perfume, & Hygiene in Ancient Egypt. Available online: https://www.ancient.eu/article/1061/cosmetics-perfume--hygiene-in-ancient-egypt/ (accessed on 4 May 2017).

Deo H T, "Eco friendly textile production", Indian Journal of Fibre & Textile Research Vol.26, March – June 2001,pp.61-73Dawkins, K. 1996. Eco-labeling: consumer's right-to-know or restrictive business practice? Minneapolis, Minn., Institute for Agriculture and Trade Policy.

Di Leva, C. E. 1998. International Environmental Law and Development. Georgetown Interna. Environ. Law Review 10 (2): 502-549.

Guerra, E.; Llompart, M.; Garcia-Jares, C. Analysis of Dyes in Cosmetics: Challenges and Recent Developments. Cosmetics 2018, 5, 47. [CrossRef]

Cosmetics Market by Category (Skin & Sun Care Products, Hair Care Products, Deodorants, Makeup & Color Cosmetics, Fragrances) and by Distribution Channel (General Departmental Store, Supermarkets,

Drug Stores, Brand Outlets)—Global Opportunity Analysis and Industry Forecast, 2014–2022. Available online: https://www.alliedmarketresearch.com/cosmetics-market (accessed on 31 July 2016).

General Introduction to the Chemistry of Dyes. Available online: https://www.ncbi.nlm.nih.gov/books/ NBK385442/ (accessed on 12 December 2010).

Economics and Management 43, 339-359.

Eiderstroem, E. 1997. Eco-labeling: Swedish Style. Forum for Applied Research in Public Policy 141(4).

Elkington, J. and Hailes, J. 1990. The green consumer guide: You can buy products that don't cost the earth. New York, Viking Press. 96p.

EMONS, W. Credence Goods and Fraudulent Experts. RAND Journal of Economics, Vol. 28 (1997), pp. 107-119.

EMONS, W. Credence Goods Monopolists. International Journal of In- dustrial Organization, Vol. 19 (2001), pp. 375-389.

European Union official website: https://ec.europa.eu/info/about-european-commission/contact_en

Feenstra, R.C. "Exact Hedonic Price Indexes," Review of Economics and Statistics 77 (1995): 634-653.

Feenstra, R.C., and J.A. Levinsohn. "Estimating Markups and Market Conduct with Multidimensional Product Attributes," Review of Economic Studies (62 (1995): 19-52.

Forest Stewardship Council: "Principles and criteria for forest stewardship" Document 1.2: <http://www.fscoax.org>

Forsyth, K. 1999. Will consumers pay more for certified wood products? Journal of Forestry 97 (2) : 18-22.

Freeman, A. M III. The Measurement of Environmental and Resource Values. Theory and Methods. Washington D.C.: Resource for the Future, 1993.

Friends of the Earth, 1993. Timber certification and eco-labeling. London, FOE:

Geetha Margret Soundri, "Ecofriendly Antimicrobial Finishing of Textiles Using Natural Extract", Journal of International Academic Research For Multidisciplinary, ISSN: 2320 – 5083, 2014, Vol 2.

Graves, P., J.C. Murdoch, M.A. Thayer, and D. Waldman. "The Robustness of Hedonic Price Estimation: Urban Air Quality," Land Economics 64(1988): 220-233.

Halvorsen, R. and R. Palmquist. "The Interpretation of Dummy Variables in Semilogarithmic Equations." American Economic Review 70:474-75 (1980).

Imhoff, Dan, and Grose, Lynda, and Carra, Roberto., "Organic Cotton Exhibit," Mimeo. Simple Life and distributed the Texas Organic Cotton Marketing Cooperative, O'Donnell, Texas (1996).

Imhoff, Dan. "Growing Pains: Organic Cotton Tests the Fibre of Growers and Manufacturers Alike," reprinted on Simple Life's web page (simplelife.com), but first printed by Farmer to Farmer, December 1995.

Incomplete Consumer Information in Laboratory Markets. Journal of Environmental labeling.

ISO 14020, ISO 14021,ISO 14024,ISO 14025, International Organization for Standardization.

Kennedy, P.E. "Estimation with Correctly Interpreted Dummy Variables in Semilogarithmic Equations," American Economic Review 71: 801 (1981).

Kirchho®, S., (2000), Green Business and Blue Angels.

Kraus, Jeff. Lab Technician at the North Carolina School of Textiles.

Labeling Issues, Policies and Practices Worldwide.

Lamport, L. 1998. The cast of (timber) certifiers: who are they? International J. Ecoforestry 11(4): 118-122.

Large Scale impoverishment of Amazonian forests by logging and fire. 1999.

Lathrop, K.W. and Centner, T.J. 1998. Eco-labeling and ISO 14000: An analysis of US regulatory systems and issues concerning adoption of type II standards. Environmental

Lee, J. et al. 1996. Trade related environmental measures; sizing and comparing impacts.

Lehtonen, Markku. 1997. Criteria in Environmental Labeling: A comparative Analysis on Environmental Criteria in Selected Labeling Schemes. Geneva, UNEP. 148p.

LIEBI, T. Trusting Labels: A Matter of Numbers? Working Paper Uni versity of Bern, No. 0201 (2002).

Lindstrom, T. 1999. Forest Certification: The View from Europe's NIPFs. Journal of Forestry 97(3): 25-31. London

Losey, J.E., Rayor, L.S. & Carter, M.E. 1999. Transgenic pollen harms monarch larvae. Nature 399 20 May): p.214.

Management 22 (2) : 163-172.

Mattoo, A. and H. V. Singh, (1994), Eco-Labelling: Policy Considera-Michaels, R. G., and V. K. Smith. "Market Segmentation And Valuing Amenities With Hedonic Models: The Case Of Hazardous Waste Sites," Journal of Urban Economics, 1990 28(2), 223-242.

Nicholson-Lord, D., (1993) 'Tis the Season to be Green, The Independent, 20 December

Nuttall, N., (1993), Shoppers can cross green products off their lists, The Times, 3 July OCDE/GD(97)105. Paris, OECD. 81p.

OECD. "Ec-labelling: Actual Effects of Selected Programmes," OCDE/GD (97) 105, 1997, Paris. (available on line at http://www.oecd.org/env/eco/books.htm#trademono)

OECD. 1997a. Case study on eco-labeling schemes. Paris, OECD (30 Dec):

OECD. 1997b. Eco-labeling: Actual Effects of Selected Programs.

Osborne, L. "Market Structure, Hedonic Models, and the Valuation of Environmental Amenities." Unpublished Ph.D. dissertation. North Carolina State University, 1995.

Osborne, L., and V. K. Smith. "Environmental Amenities, Product Differentiation, and market Power," Mimeo, 1997.

Ozanne, L.K. and Vlosky, R.P. 1996. Wood products environmental certification: the United States perspective". Forestry Chronicle 72 (2) : 157-165.

Palmquist, R. B., F. M. Roka, and T.Vukina. "Hog Operations, Environmental Effects, and Residential Property Values," Land Economics 73(1), (1997): 114-24.

Palmquist, R.B. "Hedonic Methods," in J.B Braden and C.D. Kolstad, eds. Measuring the Demand for Environmental Improvement. Amsterdam, NL: Elsevier, 1991.

Pento, T. 1997. Implementation of Public Green Procurement Programs (22-31) in Greener Purchasing: Opportunities and Innovations. Sheffield, Greenleaf Publ. 325 p.

Perloff, J. "Industrial Organization Lecture Notes," Mimeo. University of California at Berkeley (1985).

Plant, C. and Plant, J. 1991. Green business: hope or hoax? Philadelphia, New Society Publishers 136 p.

Polak, J. and Bergholm, K. 1997. Eco-labeling and trade: a cooperative approach (Jan.): Policy in a Green Market. Environmental and Resource Economics 22, 419-

Poore, M.E.D. et al. 1989. No timber without trees. London, Earthscan. 352p.

Raff, D. M.G., and M. Trajtenberg. "Quality-Adjusted Prices for the American Automobile Industry: 1906-1940." NBER Working Paper Series, Working Paper No. 5035, February 1995.

Roberts, J. T. 1998. Emerging global environment standards: prospects and perils. Journal of Developing Societies 14 (1): 144-163.

Rosen, S., "Hedonic Prices and Implicit Markets: Product Differentiation in Pure Competition." Journal of Political Economy. 82: 34-55 (1974).

Ross, B. 1997. Eco-friendly procurement training course for UN HCR. : 126 p.

Ryan, S., and Skipworth, M., (1993), Consumers turn their backs on green revolution, The Times, 4 April

Salzman, J. 1997. Informing the Green Consumer: The Debate over the Use and Abuse of Environmental Labels. Journal of Industrial Ecology 1 (2): 11-22.

Sanders, W. 1997. Environmentally Preferable Purchasing: The US Experience (946-960) in Greener Purchasing: Opportunities and Innovations. Sheffield, Greenleaf Publ. 325p.

Sayre, D. 1996. Inside ISO 14000: The competitive advantage of environmental management. Delray Beach FL., St. Lucie Press. 232p.

SHAPIRO, C. Premiums for High Quality Products as Returns to Reputa- tion. Quarterly Journal of Economics, Vol. 98, No. 4 (1983), pp. 659-680.

Stillwell, M. and van Dyke, B. 1999. An activists handbook on genetically modified organisms and the WTO. Washington DC., The Consumer's Choice Council: 20 p.

Semenzato, A.; Costantini, A.; Meloni, M.; Maramaldi, G.; Meneghin, M.; Baratto, G. Formulating O/W Emulsions with Plant-Based Actives: A Stability Challenge for an Eective Product. Cosmetics 2018, 5, 59.

Teisl, M. F., B. Roe, and R. L. Hicks. "Can Eco-labels tune a market? Evidence from dolphin-safe labeling," Presented paper at the 1997 American Agricultural Economics Association Meetings, Toronto.

THE GERSEN, C. Psychological Determinants of Paying Attention to Eco- Labels in Purchase Decisions: Model Development and Multinational Vali- dation. Journal of Consumer Policy, Vol. 23, No. 4 (2000), pp. 285-313.

Tibor, T. and Feldman, I. 1995. ISO 14000: a guide to the new environmental management standards. Burr Ridge Ill., Irwin Professional Publ. 250 p.

Torre, I. de la, & Batker, D. K. (n.d.) 1999-2000. Prawn to trade: prawn to consume. Graham WA., Industrial Shrimp Action Network (isatorre@seanet.com), [and] Asia –Pacific Townsend, M. 1998. Making things greener: motivations and influences in the greening of manufacturing. Aldershot, England, Ashgate Publisher. 203p.

U.S. Energy Information Administration, What is U.S. Electricity Generation by Energy Source?, Retrieved From: https://www.eia.gov/tools/faqs/faq.php?id=427&t=3

U.S. Energy Information Administration, Biomass Explained, Retrieved From: https://www.eia.gov/energyexplained/?page=biomass_home

U.S. Environmental Protection Agency. National Water Quality Fact Inventory: 1990 Report to Congress. EPA 503-9-92-006, Apr. 1992.

UK Eco-labelling Board website, accessed via http://www.ecosite.co.uk/Ecolabel-UK/

US Environmental Protection Agency (EPA742-R-99-001): 40 p. <www.epa.gov/opptintr/epp>

US EPA, 1993. Determinants of effectiveness for environmental certification and labeling programs. Washington, D.C., US Environmental Protect

US EPA, 1993. Status report on the use of environmental labels worldwide. Washington, D.C., US Environmental Protection Agency (742-R-93-001 September).

US EPA, 1993. The use of life-cycle assessment in environmental labeling. Washington, D.C., US Environmental Protection Agency (742-R-93-003 September).

US EPA, 1998. Environmental labeling: issues, policies, and practices worldwide. Washington DC., Environmental Protection Agency, Pollution Prevention Division Prepared by Abt

US EPA, 1999. Comprehensive procurement guidelines (CPG) program. Washington, D.C., US Environmental Protection Agency: <www.epa.gov/cpg>

US EPA, 1999. Environmentally preferable purchasing program: Private sector pioneers: How companies are incorporating environmentally preferable purchases. Washington, D.C.,

USG, 1993. Federal acquisition, recycling, and waste prevention. Washington DC., Executive Order: (20 October).

USG, 1998. Greening the government through waste prevention, recycling, and federal acquisition. Washington, D.C., Executive Order 13101 (September).

Kijjoa, A.; Sawangwong, P. Drugs and Cosmetics from the Sea. Mar. Drugs 2004, 2, 73–82. [CrossRef]

Wang, J.; Pan, L.; Wu, S.; Lu, L.; Xu, Y.; Zhu, Y.; Guo, M.; Zhuang, S. Recent Advances on Endocrine Disrupting Eects of UV Filters. Int. J. Environ. Res. Public Health 2016, 13, 782.

Bilal, A.I.; Tilahun, Z.; Shimels, T.; Gelan, Y.B.; Osman, E.D. Cosmetics Utilization Practice in Jigjiga Town, Eastern Ethiopia: A Community Based Cross-Sectional Study. Cosmetics 2016, 3, 40.

Ting, C.T.; Hsieh, C.M.; Chang, H.-P.; Chen, H.-S. Environmental Consciousness and Green Customer Behavior: The Moderating Roles of Incentive Mechanisms. Sustainability 2019, 11, 819.

Chen, K.; Deng, T. Research on the Green Purchase Intentions from the Perspective of Product Knowledge. Sustainability 2016, 8, 943.

Wang, H.; Ma, B.; Bai, R. How Does Green Product Knowledge Eectively Promote Green Purchase Intention? Sustainability 2019, 11, 1193.

Nguyen, T.T.H.; Yang, Z.; Nguyen, N.; Johnson, L.W.; Cao, T.K. Greenwash and Green Purchase Intention: The Mediating Role of Green Skepticism. Sustainability 2019, 11, 2653.

Cinelli, P.; Coltelli, M.B.; Signori, F.; Morganti, P.; Lazzeri, A. Cosmetic Packaging to Save the Environment: Future Perspectives. Cosmetics 2019, 6, 26.

Eixarch, H.; Wyness, L.; Siband, M. The Regulation of Personalized Cosmetics in the EU. Cosmetics 2019, 6, 29.

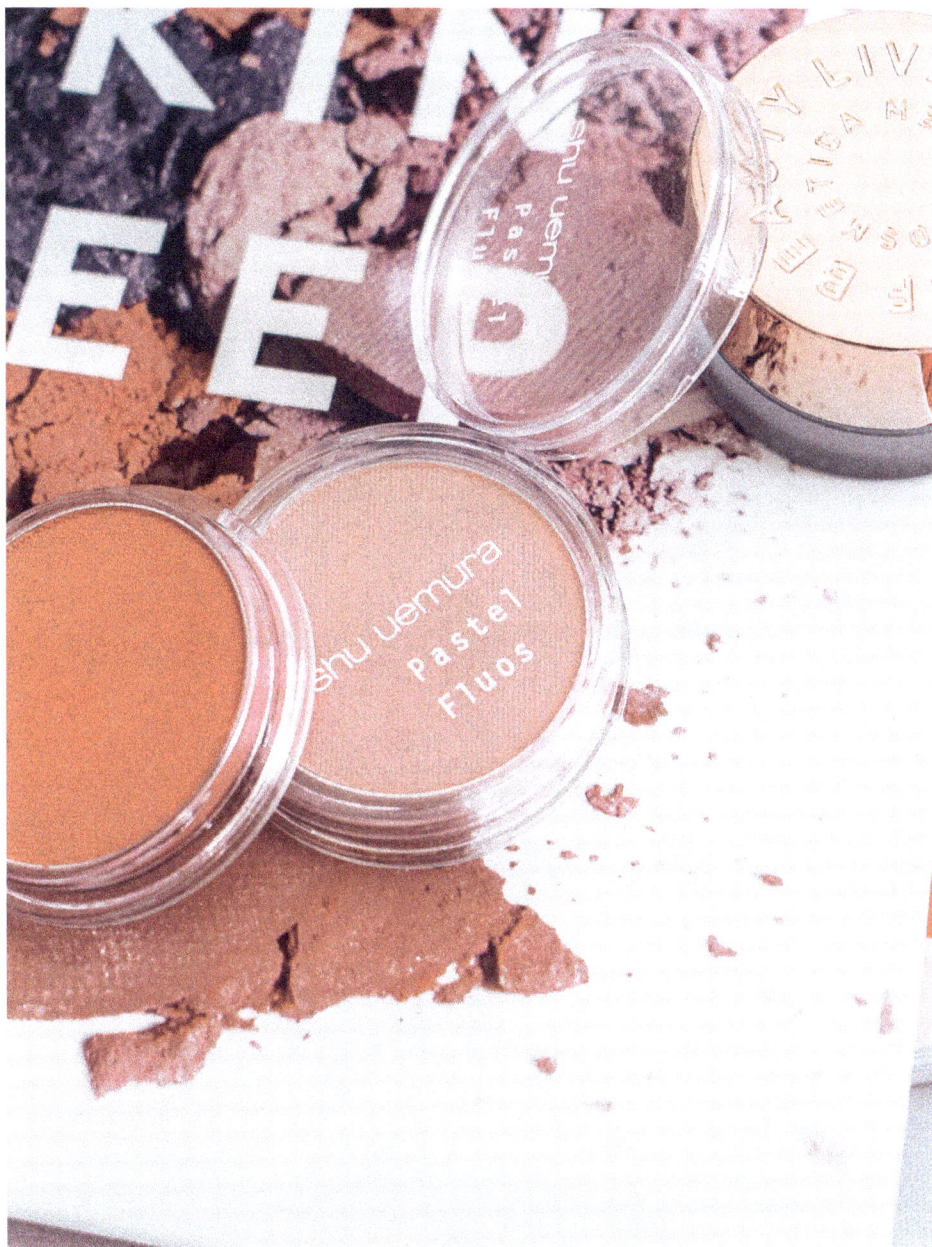

APPENDIX I: SEARCH BY LOGOS

H ere you can search the logos in this volume. It will help you to better undersand the Ecolabels you may encounter while shopping. Buying Eco-products will aid in having a better environment with minimum polution during production processes. Three important parameteres for shopping are **quality**, **price** & **environmental impacts** of the products.

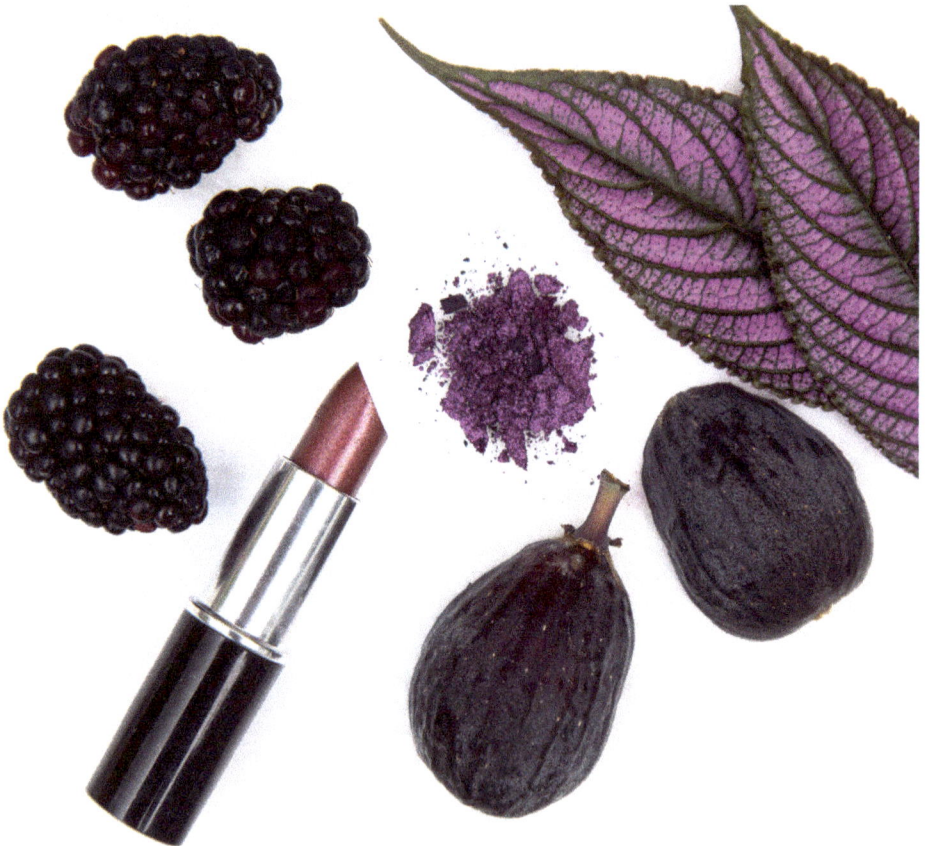

Vol.4 Goto page: 29	Vol.4 Goto page: 44
Vol.4 Goto page: 50	Vol.4 Goto page: 81
Vol.4 Goto page: 58	Vol.4 Goto page: 58
Vol.4 Goto page: 58	Vol.4 Goto page: 40

Vol.4 Goto page: 35	Vol.4 Goto page: 37
Vol.4 Goto page: 44	Vol.4 Goto page: 32
Vol.4 Goto page: 38	Vol.4 Goto page: 32
Vol.4 Goto page: 42 ,41	Vol.4 Goto page: 43

VEGAN	PARABEN FREE
Vol.4 Goto page: 72	Vol.4 Goto page: 44
sustainable florist	NITRATES FREE
Vol.4 Goto page: 39	Vol.4 Goto page: 72
NOT TESTED ON ANIMALS	SULFATEN FREE
Vol.4 Goto page: 72	Vol.4 Goto page: 72
WITHOUT GMO	ORGANIC COSMETICS
Vol.4 Goto page: 72	Vol.4 Goto page: 72

FRESH COSMETICS	ORGANIC CERTIFICATION
Vol.4 Goto page: 72	Vol.4 Goto page: 36
SODIUM FREE	
Vol.4 Goto page: 72	Vol.4 Goto page: 34
Vol.4 Goto page: 31	Vol.4 Goto page: 30
Vol.4 Goto page: 33	Vol.4 Goto page: 37

Sustainable Health and Beauty with Algae

Ingredients that come from marine creatures and algae are also found in many cosmetics. Many biologically active materials that can be used for cosmetic purposes can be extracted from marine lifeforms. Such as algae (macro- and micro-algae) as a prime example. Their usage in cosmetic products can be accredited to their skincare attributes. Algae hydrate the skin, aid circulation, activate the renewal and metabolism of cells, regulate the operation of sebaceous glands, regenerate tissue, have an anti-inflammatory eect, and increase skin resistance. Bio-active ingredients coming from natural sources have a well-known positive effect in cosmetic usage, which also serve as incentive for consumers.

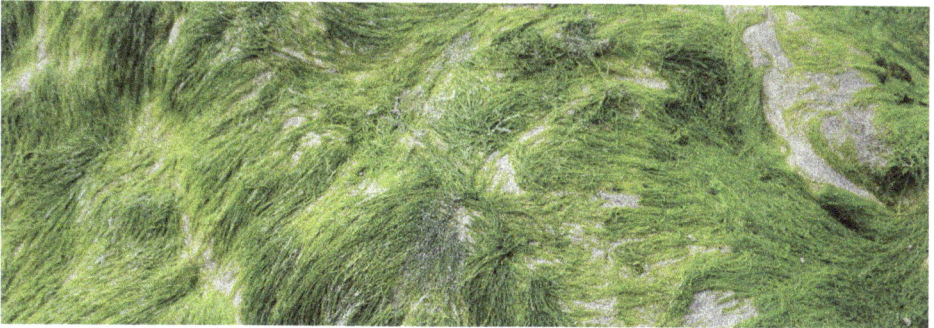

Of these, gallotannins have a very intriguing potential. Caeic acid (CAF) is one of the most promising active ingredients, since it is an anti-oxidant, anti-inflammatory, and anti-wrinkle as well. In case of local usage, increasing its biological availability may lead to source material expecting new cosmetic interest. Clay minerals also have exceptional qualities, among others, low or no toxicity, and high bio-compatibility.

Environmental Friendly Photos

Environmental friendly photos will be placed in this appendix. These photos can be received in the Top Ten Award International Network inbox from anywhere and everywhere, all over the globe. You can send your appropriate photos to us for them to be considered for publishing in one of the future, related volumes. They will be published with proper credit to the sender. The pictures can also be images of the Ecolabels existing in products within your country.

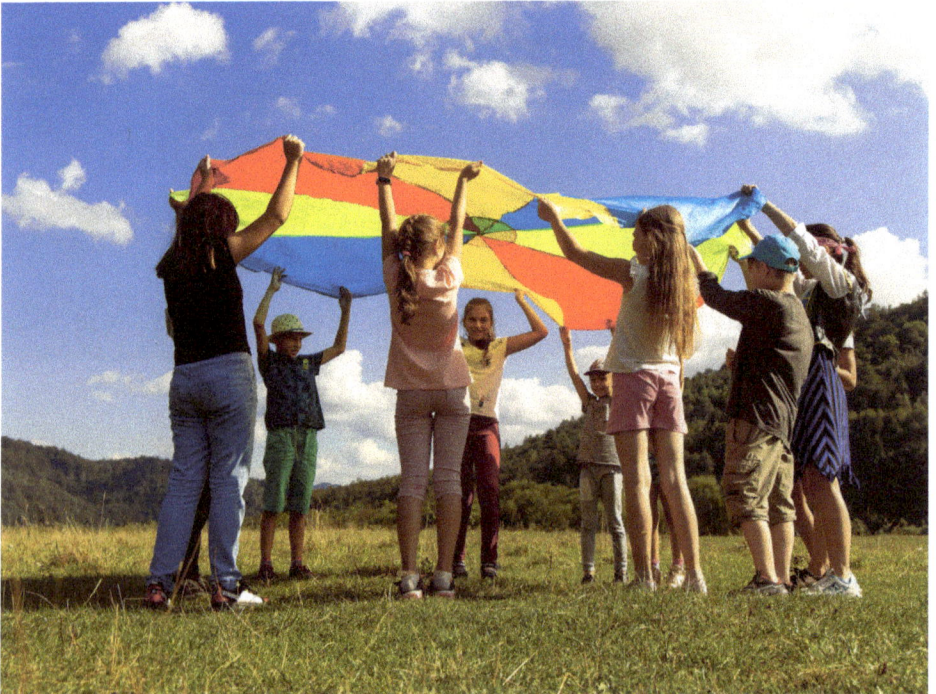

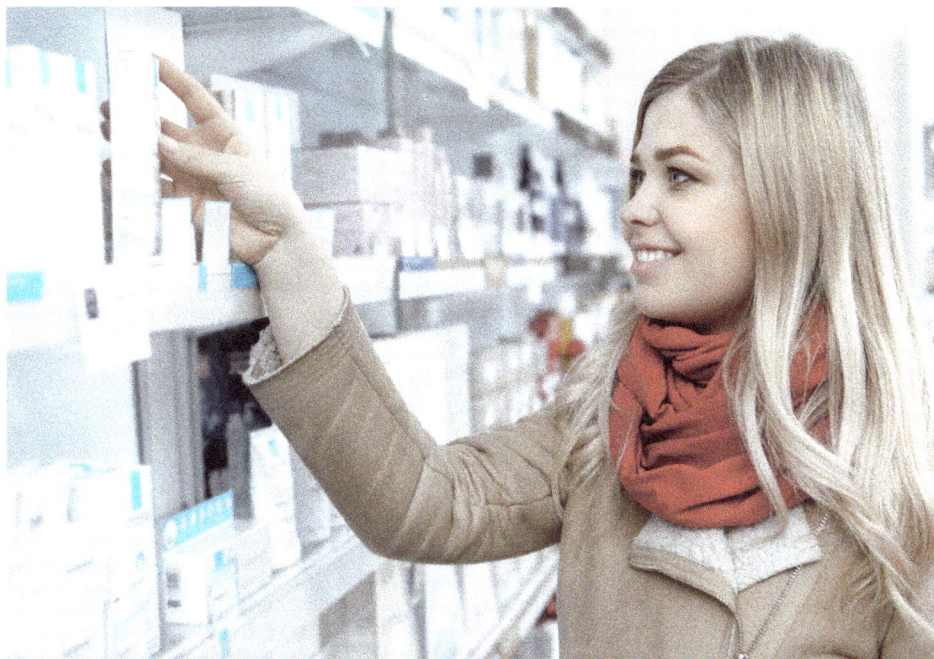

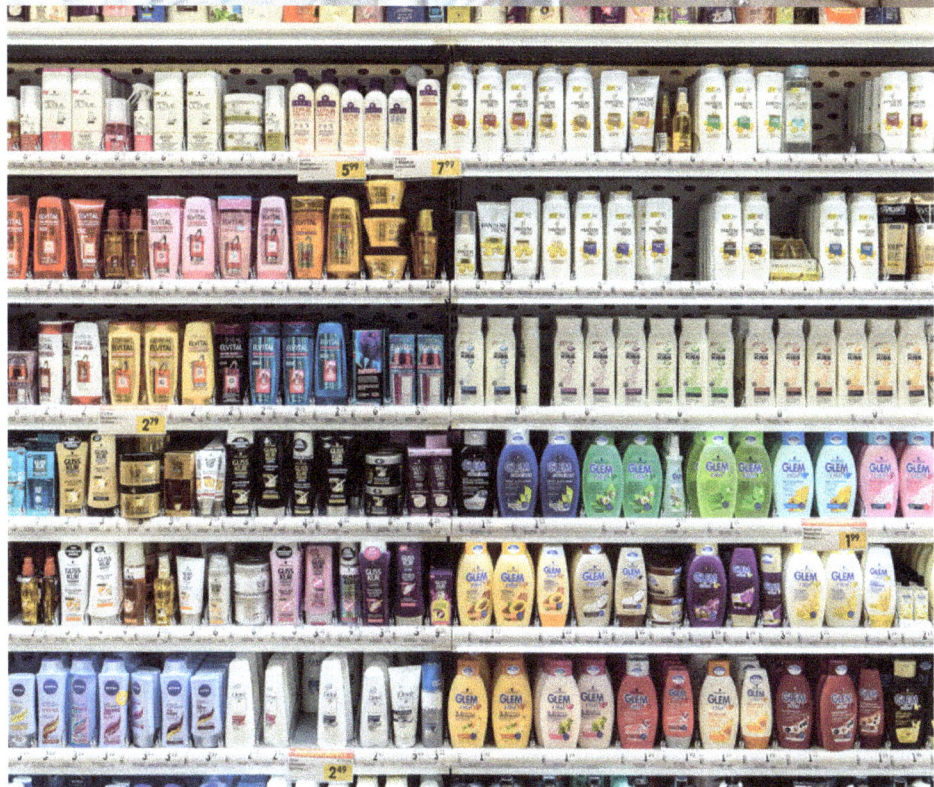

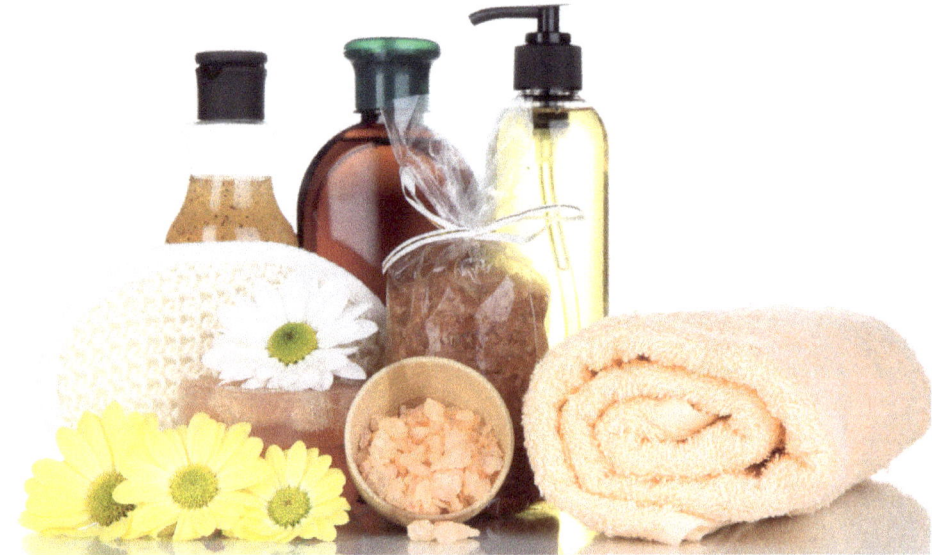

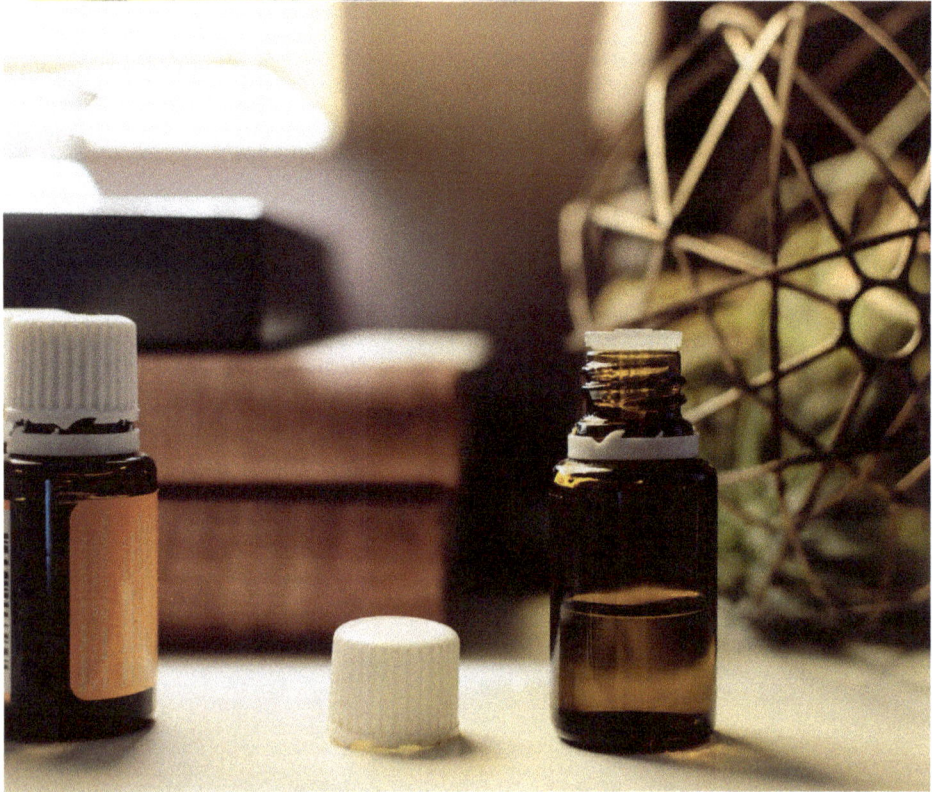

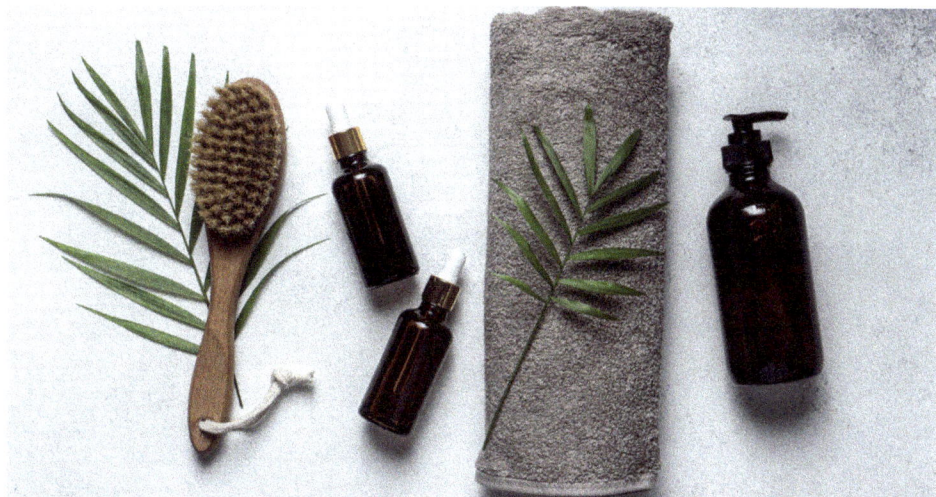

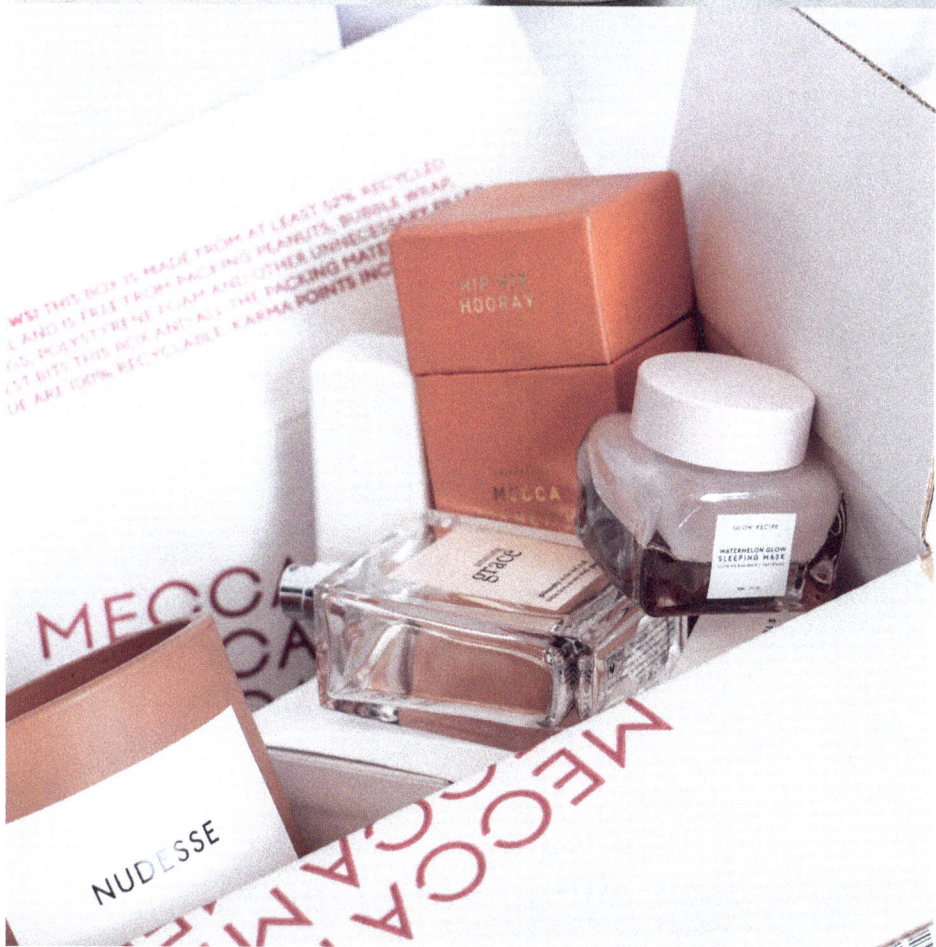

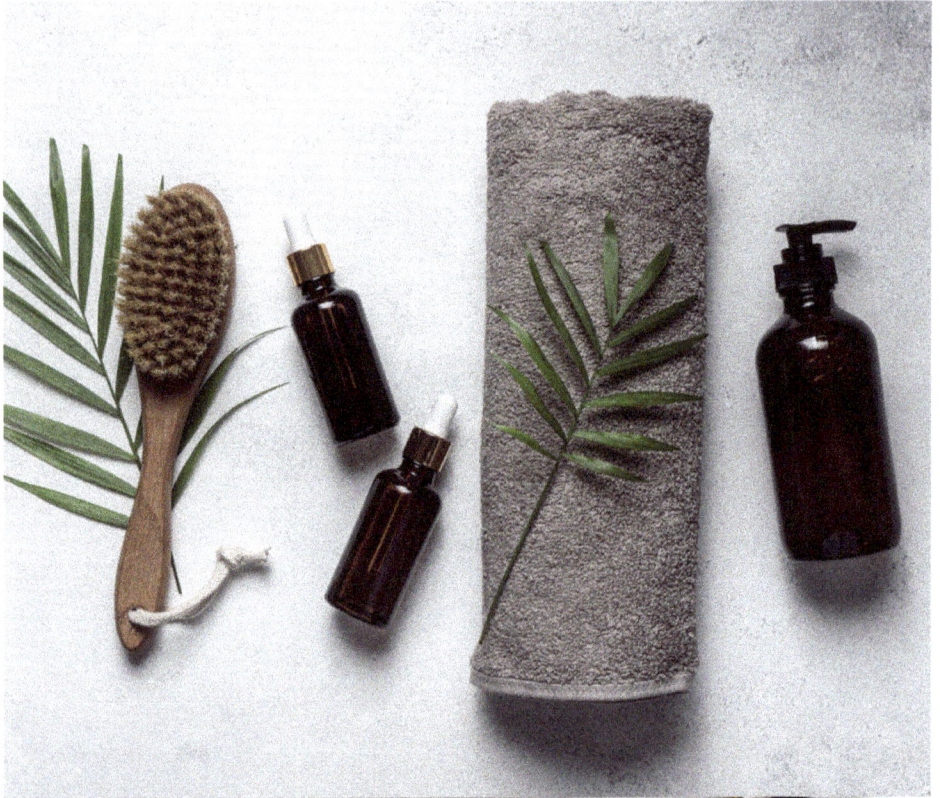

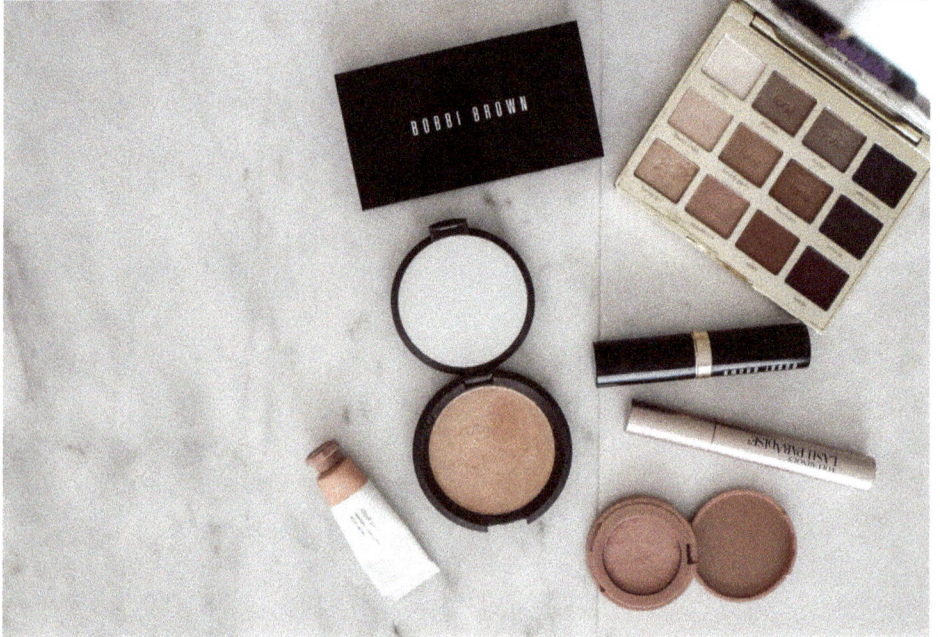

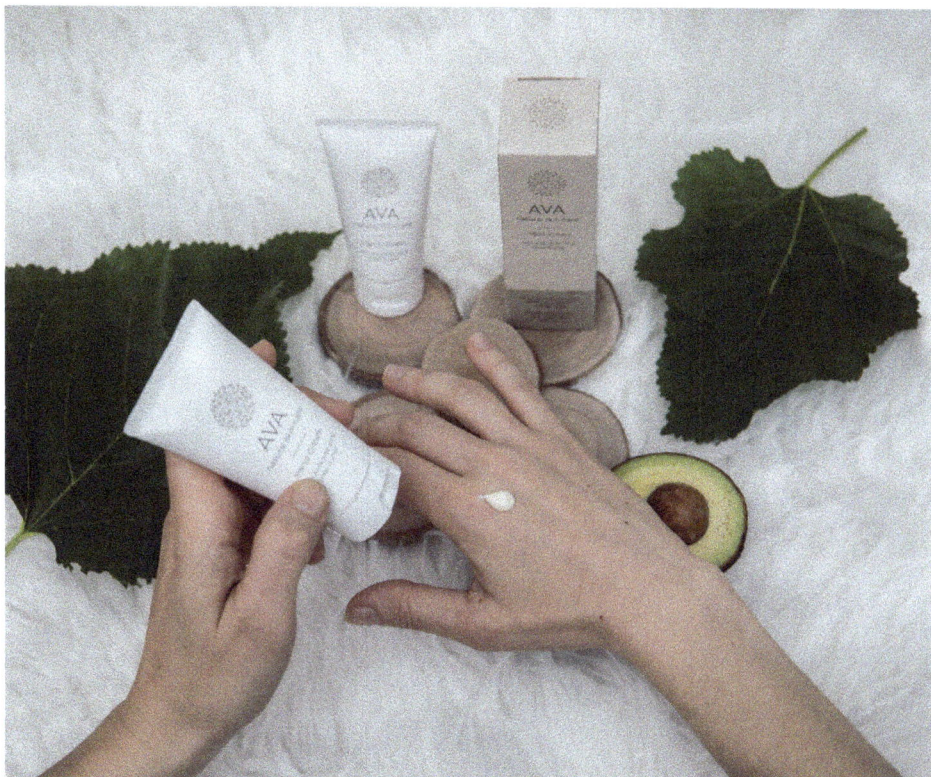

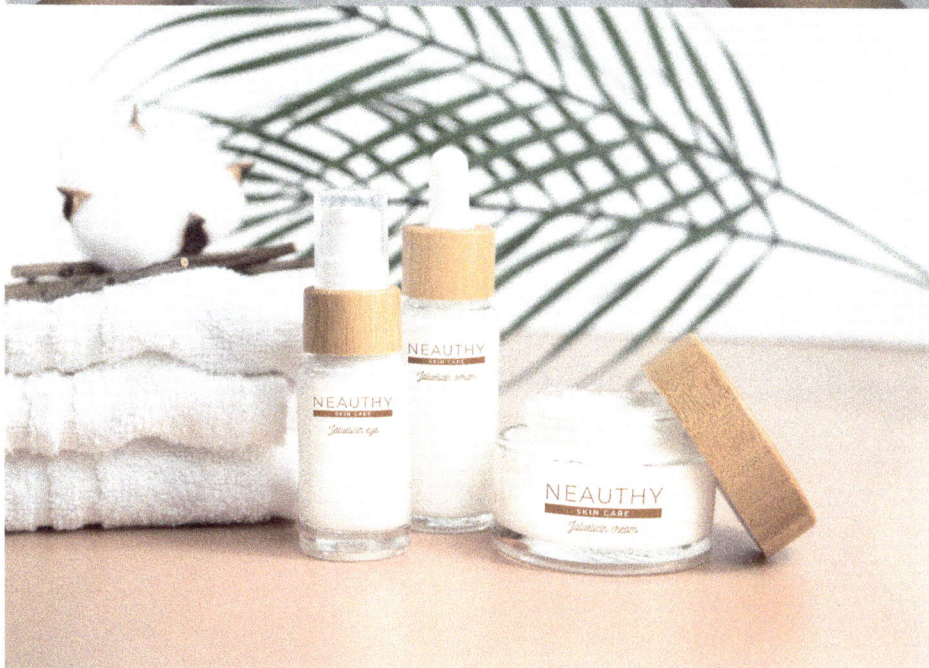

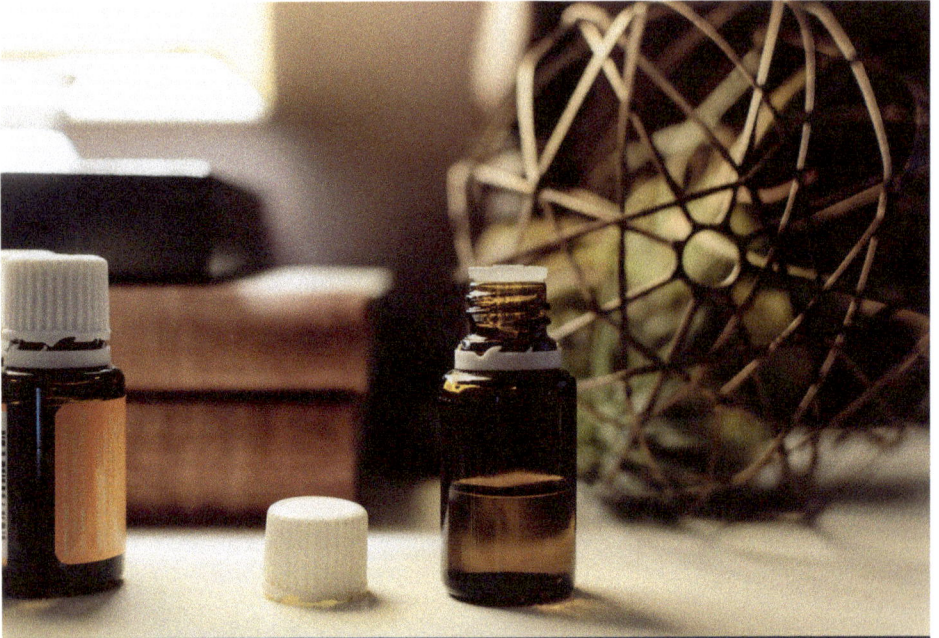

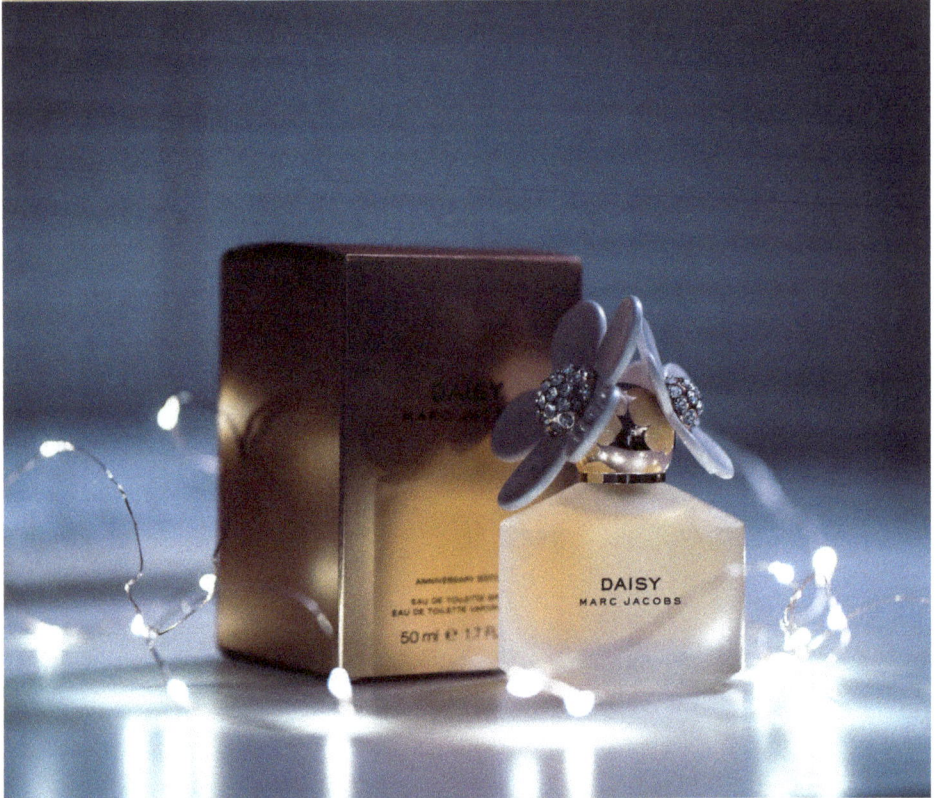

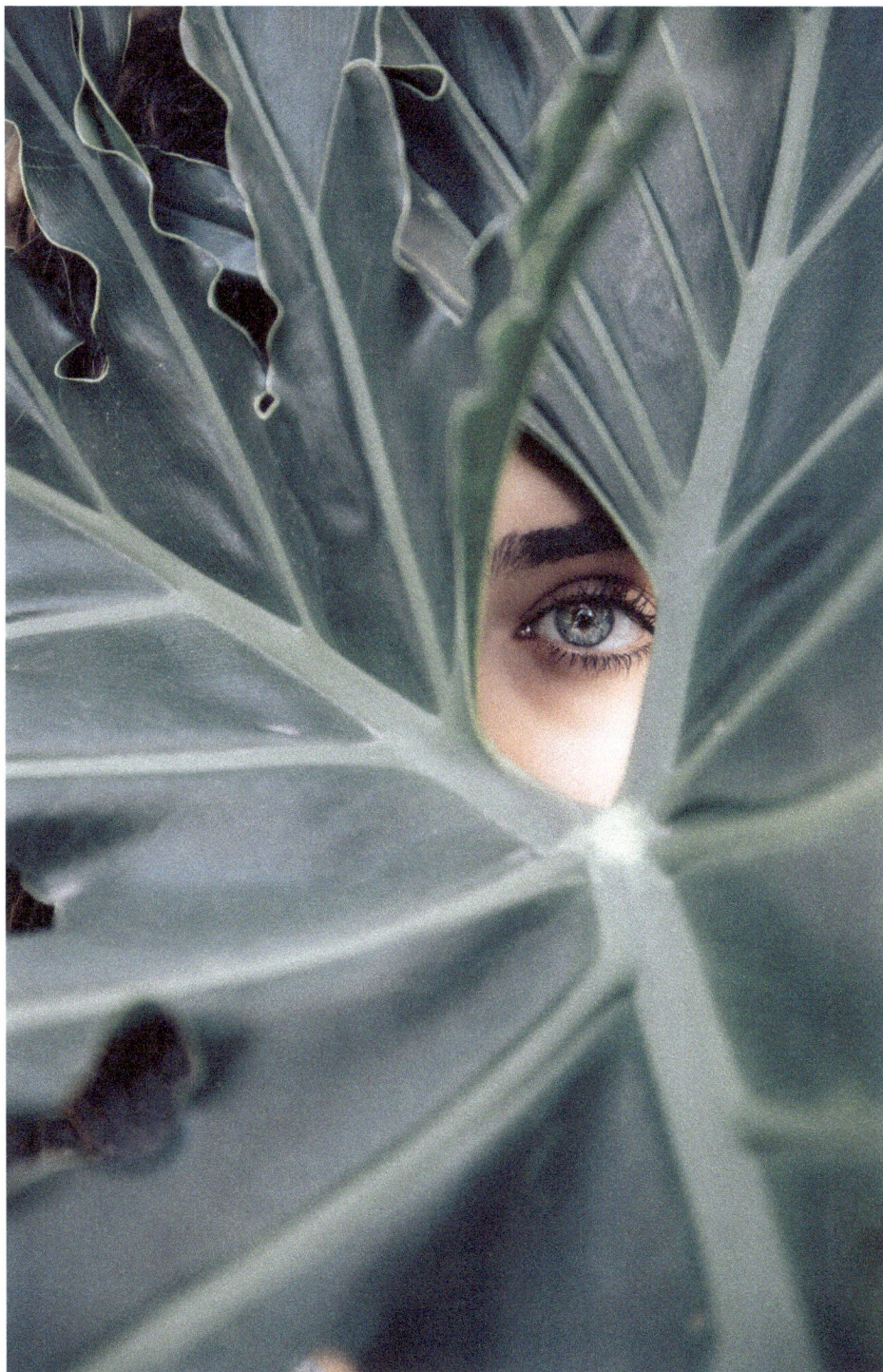

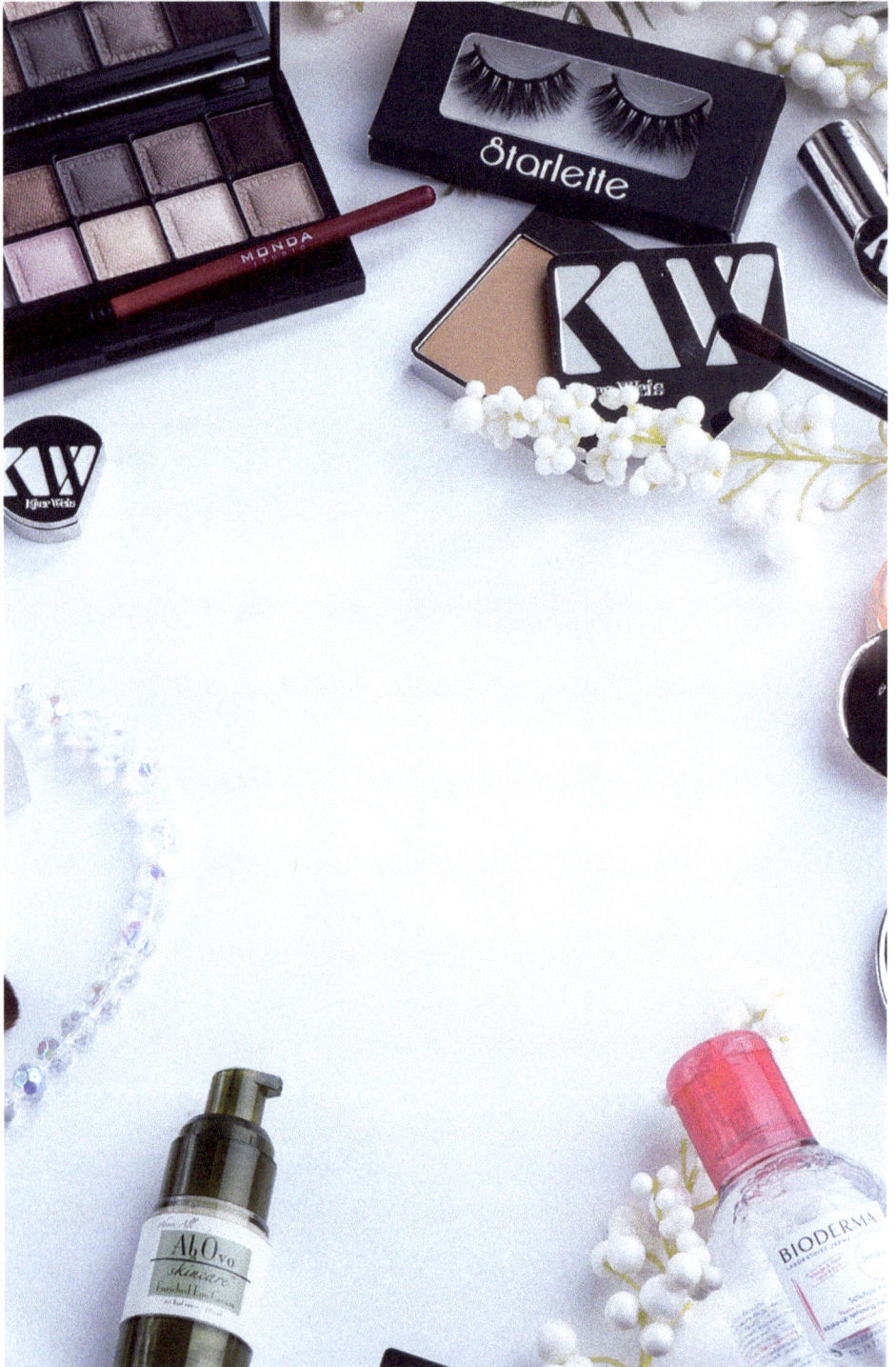

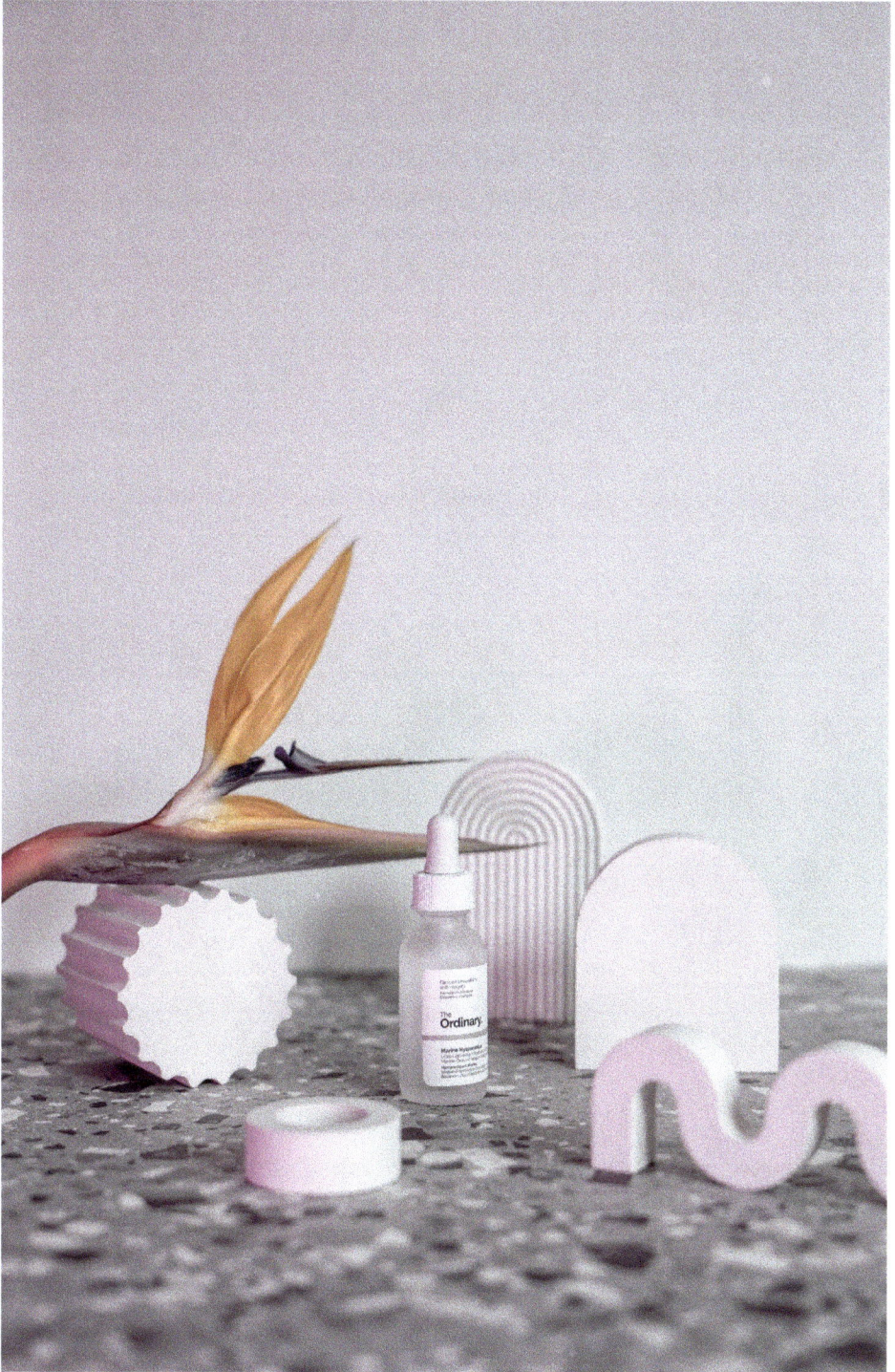

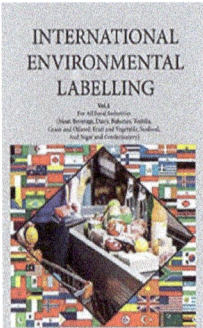

Vol.1

For All People who wish to take care of Climate Change,
Food Industries:
(Meat, Beverage, Dairy, Bakeries, Tortilla,
Grain and Oilseed, Fruit and Vegetable, Seafood,
And Sugar and Confectionery)

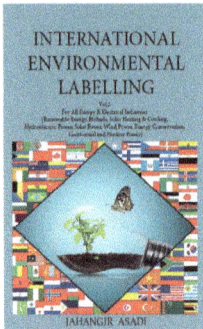

Vol.2

For All People who wish to take care of Climate Change,
Electrical Industries:
(Renewable Energy, Biofuels, Solar Heating
& Cooling, Hydroelectric Power, Solar Power,
Wind Power, Energy Conservation, Geothermal
and Nuclear Power)

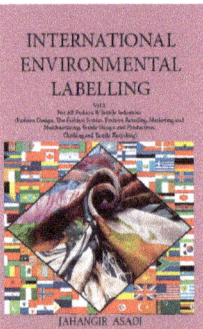

Vol.3

For All People who wish to take care of Climate Change,
Fashion & Textile Industries:
(Fashion Design, The Fashion System, Fashion
Retailing, Marketing and Marchandizing, Textile
Design and Production, Clothing and
Textile Recycling)

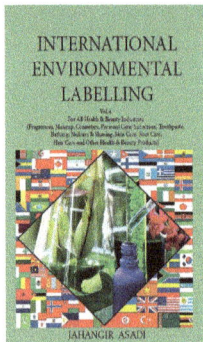

Vol.4

For All People who wish to take care of Climate Change,
Health & Beauty Industries:
(Fragrances, Makeup, Cosmetics, Personal Care,
Sunscreen, Toothpaste, Bathing, Nailcare &
Shaving, Skin Care, Foot Care, Hair Care and
Other Health & Beauty Products)

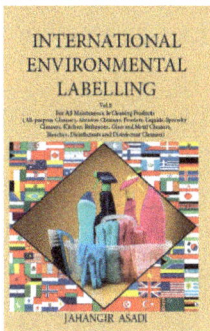

Vol.5

For All People who wish to take care of Climate Change,
Maintenance & Cleaning Products:
(All-purpose Cleaners, Abrasive Cleaners,
Powders. Liquids, Specialty Cleaners, Kitchen,
Bathroom, Glass and Metal Cleaners, Bleaches,
Disinfectants and Disinfectant Cleaners)

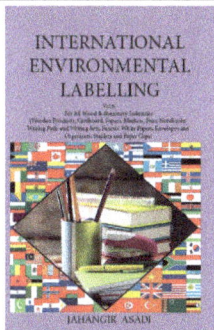

Vol.6

For All People who wish to take care of Climate Change,
Wood & Stationery Industries:
(Wooden Products, Cardboard, Papers, Markers,
Pens, NoteBooks, Writing Pads and Writing Sets,
Pencils, White Papers, Envelopes and
Organizers, Staplers and Paper Clips)

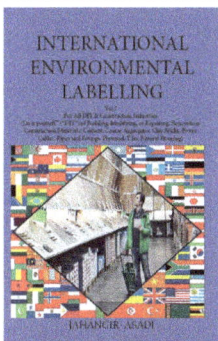

Vol.7

For All People who wish to take care of Climate Change,
DIY & Construction Industries:
(Do it yourself " ("DIY") of Building, Modifying,
or Repairing, Renovation, Construction
Materials, Cement, Coarse Aggregates. Clay
Bricks, Power Cables, Pipes and Fittings,
Plywood, Tiles, Natural Flooring)

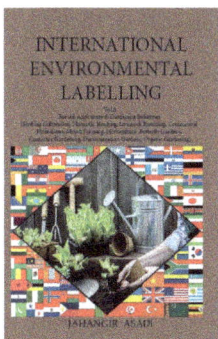

Vol.8

For All People who wish to take care of Climate Change,
Agricuture & Gardening Industries:
(Shifting Cultivation, Nomadic Herding,
Livestock Ranching, Commercial Plantations,
Mixed Farming, Horticulture, Butterfly Gardens,
Container Gardening, Demonstration Gardens,
Organic Gardening)

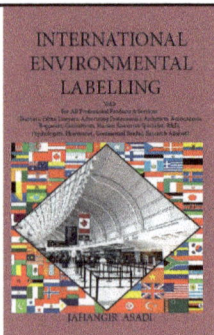

INTERNATIONAL ENVIRONMENTAL LABELLING Vol.9 *For All Professional Products & Services* JAHANGIR ASADI	# Vol.9 For All People who wish to take care of Climate Change, Professional Products & Services: (Teachers, Pilots, Lawyers, Advertising Professionals, Architects, Accountants, Engineers, Consultants, Human Resources Specialist, R&D, Psychologists, Pharmacist, Commercial Banker, Research Analyst)
INTERNATIONAL ENVIRONMENTAL LABELLING Vol.10 *For All Financial Products & Services* JAHANGIR ASADI	# Vol.10 For All People who wish to take care of Climate Change, Financial Products & Services: (Banking, Professional Advisory, Wealth Management, Mutual Funds, Insurance, Stock Market, Treasury/Debt Instruments, Tax/Audit Consulting, Capital Restructuring, Portfolio Management)
INTERNATIONAL ENVIRONMENTAL LABELLING Vol.11 *For All Tourism Industries* JAHANGIR ASADI	# Vol.11 For All People who wish to take care of Climate Change, Tourism Industries: (Airline Industry, Travel Agent, Car Rental, Water Transport, Coach Services, Railway, Spacecraft, Hotels, Shared Accommodation, Camping, Bed & Breakfast, Cruises, Tour Operators)
INTERNATIONAL ENVIRONMENTAL LABELLING Knowledge Test for Vol.1 to Vol.11 For all Schools and Libraries Knowledge Test JAHANGIR ASADI	## Set Box Books Vol.1-11 ## + Free Knowledge Test ### for **Schools, Libraries, Homes and Offices all over the globe:** **www.TopTenAward.Net**

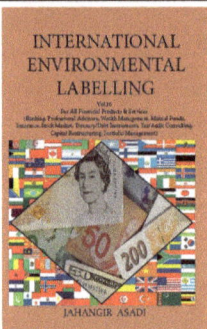

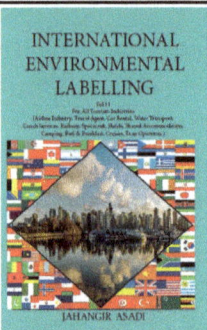

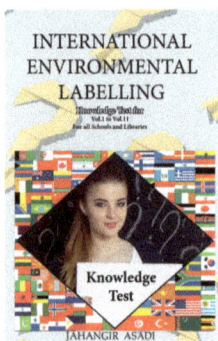

www.ingramcontent.com/pod-product-compliance
Lightning Source LLC
Chambersburg PA
CBHW041217030426

42336CB00023B/3368